Revertigo

Terrace Books, a trade imprint of the University of Wisconsin Press, takes its name from the Memorial Union Terrace, located at the University of Wisconsin–Madison. Since its inception in 1907, the Wisconsin Union has provided a venue for students, faculty, staff, and alumni to debate art, music, politics, and the issues of the day. It is a place where theater, music, drama, literature, dance, outdoor activities, and major speakers are made available to the campus and the community. To learn more about the Union, visit www.union.wisc.edu.

REVERTIGO

An Off-Kilter Memoir

FLOYD SKLOOT

Terrace Books

A trade imprint of the University of Wisconsin Press

Terrace Books
A trade imprint of the University of Wisconsin Press
1930 Monroe Street, 3rd Floor
Madison, Wisconsin 53711-2059
uwpress.wisc.edu

3 Henrietta Street
London WC2E 8LU, England
eurospanbookstore.com

Printed in the United States of America

Library of Congress Cataloging-in-Publication Data

Skloot, Floyd, author.
Revertigo: an off-kilter memoir / Floyd Skloot.
pages   cm
ISBN 978-0-299-29950-7 (cloth: alk. paper)
ISBN 978-0-299-29953-8 (e-book)
I. Skloot, Floyd.   2. Authors, American—20th century—Biography.
3. Authors, American—21st century—Biography.   I. Title.
PS3569.K577Z46   2014
818'.54—dc23
[B]
2013028359

For Beverly

His dizzy brain spun fast,
And down he sunk.

George Gordon, Lord Byron,

from *Don Juan*, Canto II, 110

Contents

Acknowledgments

Chapters of *Revertigo: An Off-Kilter Memoir* originally appeared in the following publications, sometimes in different versions. I thank the editors for their support of my work:

> *Boulevard*: "Anniversary Fever," "Beep Beep," "Revertigo," and "To Land's End and Back: A 1,512-Mile Drive Around Southern England"
> *Colorado Review*: "The Famous Recipe"
> *Ecotone*: "Sway Me Smooth: Soundtrack for an MRI of the Brain"
> *Harvard Review*: "Playing the Cock"
> *Post Road*: "Elliptical Journey"
> *Prairie Schooner*: "Something to Marvel At: Discovering Jules Verne at Sixty"
> *The Seneca Review*: "The Side Effect of Side Effects"
> *The Sewanee Review*: "The Bottom Shelf: On Novels I Keep Trying and Failing to Read" and "The Top Shelf: On Books I Need Beside Me"
> *Southwest Review*: "Senior Speech" and "Some Things Nearly So, Others Nearly Not: *The King and I* and Me"

"The Famous Recipe" was reprinted in *Best Food Writing 2011*. "Senior Speech" was cited as a Notable Essay of 2009 in *The Best American*

Essays 2010 and for Special Mention in *The Pushcart Prize XXXIV*, 2010. "The Bottom Shelf: On Novels I Keep Trying and Failing to Read" was cited as a Notable Essay of 2010 in *The Best American Essays 2011*. "Something to Marvel At: Discovering Jules Verne at Sixty" was cited as Notable Nonrequired Reading of 2010 in *The Best American Nonrequired Reading 2011*. "Revertigo" was cited as a Notable Essay of 2011 in *The Best American Essays 2012*. "Sway Me Smooth: Soundtrack for an MRI of the Brain" was cited for Special Mention in *The Pushcart Prize XXXVI*, 2012.

In the six years it took to write *Revertigo: An Off-Kilter Memoir*, my wife, Beverly Hallberg, helped keep me balanced. When that wasn't enough, she held me still in a spinning world. She also read drafts of each chapter, and thought things through with me. My daughter, Rebecca Skloot, inspired me—and millions of readers—with her brilliant work, insight, courage, and passion for truth. I'm grateful to Kerry and Nigel Arkell for their gustatory bravery, Dr. Doug Beers for decades of masterful medical care, Andrew Blauner for his good faith, George Core for the walking stick, Joan Katz for my mother's recipe, Guohui Liu for releasing the wind, and Hilda Raz for the flying advice.

Revertigo

PROLOGUE

On Ross Island, across the Willamette from our home at river mile fourteen, there's a great blue heron rookery in the upper limbs of some cottonwood trees. Beverly and I love to watch these enormous birds, some of them four feet tall and weighing nearly eight pounds, as they gather at their nests, circling and landing or taking off from the slenderest branches.

It seems astounding to me that creatures so hulking can maintain their places up there as the wind blows, as the rains fall. When I see them at their most eloquently poised, when everything they're holding onto is swaying and swirling, I usually lose my balance, which is why I make sure to sit while watching them.

ⓢ

At the center of *Revertigo: An Off-Kilter Memoir* is an attack of un-relenting vertigo that began—out of nowhere—on the morning of March 27, 2009, and ended on the evening of August 12, 2009, as suddenly as it had begun. Those 138 days seemed so anomalous, such a weird and isolated period in my life.

As I began writing about it, I realized it would make no sense—or rather that it would seem to make too much apparent sense—if I told the story in a traditionally structured, conventional memoir. When you're not in perfect balance, when body and world are askew, everything familiar is transformed. There's a destabilizing of the self and its encounter with the world, a whirling of space and time. Nothing is ever still. Topsy-turvy rules. To capture what it felt like to be unceasingly vertiginous would require a matching off-kilterness of form, a structure that was tenuous, shifting, unpredictable.

I also realized that, for the previous three years, I'd already been writing this book. My work was exploring balance and its loss, how the forces of uncertainty and sudden change and displacement had shaped me since childhood, as it shapes many of us, by repeatedly knocking me awry, requiring me to react and adapt fast, urgently re-align my hopes and plans, even my perceptions. It seemed as though my life, and my writing about my life, had been preparing me for just such a time of radical off-kilterness. I kept waiting for the book to orient itself in the usual way, only to find that disorientation was its dominant mode.

Looked at as a weird and isolated period in my life, the 138 days of vertigo were one thing, with a beginning and end, and I needed to take that look. But I came to understand that there was more to the story. For instance, there was something inaccurate in the whole notion of *beginning and end* as having finite form. I realized that the shape of this book needed to be open, not linear, and not static.

ᔐ

I wasn't going to have a problem. It had been almost eight months since my vertigo had vanished, and I was walking fine. No cane, no stumbling or grabbing onto stationary objects for balance, no neck-and-shoulder-locked gait. Very little swooning. Swooning only occurred when—as happens to many people—I did something like look up at the clouds while walking. Yes, I was back to almost normal. Except there were maybe a few oddities, such as getting light-headed when I merely thought about riding on Portland's aerial tram, swaying as it rises five hundred feet during its three-minute trip from the south waterfront up to Oregon Health and Science University's main campus. Or when I saw a still photograph of lions veering in pursuit of a zebra. Or that one time when a lightbulb flickered. Odd, okay, but truly I was back in balance. Recovered. No longer vertiginous.

So it never crossed my mind to worry about going to look at riverfront condo units that were set for auction in early April. Beverly and I had decided to sell our home, abandon stairs and roof maintenance and yard work and tree trimming, all the things I'd be unable to do again if vertigo recurred. Simplify, keep level.

The first building we were looking at was a thirty-one-story, elliptical-shaped glass tower looming 325 feet above the Willamette River. This was going to be great. And it was, as we got off the elevator on the twenty-seventh floor and entered the unit being used as a temporary auction office. Then I encountered the view and began reeling, trying to brace myself against a desk, a kitchen island, an interior wall. I seemed more like a drunk than a prospective buyer.

It took us a subsequent month to determine that I was all right, that I could be comfortable and stable, only up to the sixth floor of a condo. And provided I didn't go outside on the balcony. And as long as I held on to something when I stood against the interior glass walls and looked down. So now we live on the sixth floor of a twenty-one-story building at the river's edge, and I can *sit* by the window and watch boats, even speedboats, race by. I can watch herons. I'm post-vertigo, except when I'm not, for three years, ten months, and twenty-four days.

§

If I can't even be sure that my apparently self-contained episode of vertigo has truly ended, then I don't want to write a memoir about it that embodies traditional notions of balance, flow, imposed logic, closure. And if the apparently self-contained episode helps me understand that vertiginousness has always been a central part of my life, and that I was writing about it even before the attack happened, preparing for it, then I want this book to reflect just such narrative and structural fluidity, underscoring that where you find yourself is always contingent. I want the reader to join, through the book's formal arrangement, in the process of finding and losing and refinding balance.

Revertigo: An Off-Kilter Memoir follows a loose chronological sequence from adolescence (the first chapter takes place shortly before my thirteenth birthday) to the onset of senior citizenship (the last chapters take place as I reached sixty-five). Part One, "O Wondrous Transformation!," is concerned with the volatile forces that shaped and reshaped me as I first sought to claim some sort of stable identity. Mine was not a world of fixed principles, firm beliefs, trustworthy foundations. It was a mercurial, eruptive, shape-shifting place, theatrical and often melodramatic, full of sudden harm, changes of fortune, changes of character. I never felt firmly grounded to the earth or connected to those around me, who so often seemed to morph into someone else. I was the son of a faux aristocrat and a chicken butcher. I learned about love through musical comedy lyrics, didn't sound the way I wanted to, was a boy who didn't care about cars. It was fitting that my adolescence was spent on a sandy island. In Part One, I do everything I can to find my role in a play whose story and structure make no sense to me, and learn to express myself with some kind of integrity.

Part Two, "On and Off the Page," follows my immersion in—okay, my obsession with—literature. With reading and acting and writing, with finding myself within the pages of books, with the way literature infuses my daily life, so that a walk in the woods becomes a chapter in a Jules Verne novel. But even there, in an obvious quest for understanding, meaning, coherence (if I read enough, I will learn how the world works, how it holds together), things keep changing on me. My sense of myself as expressed in what I read, or in what I discover as I write, is full of surprise turns for me, revelations and contradictions. I often find my response to books is off-kilter, far from canonical opinion, far from what I expected. Though it doesn't contain all the answers, literature—and the real-life love story I'm living with Beverly—has come to serve as my balance pole. If that balance pole occasionally throws me off balance, I feel I'm better off for that.

Part Three, "A Spinning World," deals with the attack of vertigo. It also deals with learning to live with the long-term, life-changing illness that came before and continues after the attack of vertigo. With trying to make sense of it and take control of how I manage my health. The book's final section, "Cartwheels on the Moon," deals with a trio of tenuous, postvertigo-but-dizzying journeys to real places, Spain and England, and to a place known only in my mother's unhinged fantasies, somewhere near the junction of France, Italy, Russia, and Long Beach, New York.

And this prologue is actually an epilogue.

Part One

O WONDROUS TRANSFORMATION!

But, O Wondrous Transformation!

Henry Wadsworth Longfellow

from *The Song of Hiawatha*

1

SOME THINGS NEARLY SO, OTHERS NEARLY NOT

The King and I *and Me*

Is a puzzlement!

Mildred was a deeply disturbing King. Tall and full bodied, with cascading curly blonde hair, she wore cat's-eye glasses, vivid crimson lipstick, and a cubist smile. She ordered people around, then giggled at herself. Her autocratic fists-on-hips stance looked unsettlingly come-hither, even when she donned her bald headpiece. She came across like Phil Silvers being played by Lucille Ball.

I knew Mildred as Mrs. Levine, my friend Richard's mother, a long-lashed and hip-swaying dancer at bar mitzvahs, key player in my mother's mah-jongg group, giver of ballyhooed dinner parties with her husband, Vance. She specialized in cream cheese and grape jelly sandwiches on pumpernickel hacked into erratic triangles. But she was also the director of our local community theater, and for its spring 1960 production of *The King and I,* the classic Rodgers and Hammerstein musical about a Welsh woman who becomes tutor and governess to the king of Siam's children, Mildred had cast herself as the tyrannical and fickle King Mongkut, Rama IV, husband of twenty-three wives and father of sixty-seven princes and princesses. It was the arrogant potentate's role made famous by a shaven-headed baritone named Yul Brynner, former circus acrobat and nightclub singer.

During early rehearsals, Mildred still looked like herself and still behaved like herself, only a little bossier. As the play's director, she would sit near the aisle of the auditorium's middle row, head wreathed in smoke from her Lucky Strikes, and issue critiques or instructions. Then she would run up to the stage and, in character as the King, glower and pose between her lines. But she spoke those lines with a dampened soprano rasp, and seemed more petulant than regal, stamping her foot to convey his emphatic style. There was no one to critique her performance and, sometimes, she would berate herself using her Mongkut voice. Once, speaking Anna's lines instead of her own, then speaking her own instead of Anna's, she shook her head and burst into tears.

To a boy nearing thirteen, playing one of Mildred/Mongkut's sons, this was all elusive and muddling. In the back of the auditorium, doing my homework with the other royal children, I had serious trouble with focus. Morphing Mildred was a lot to keep track of.

So were my new feelings toward one of the other royal children, red-headed Jacqueline, who was required to hold my hand as we marched onstage together and sit next to me in our classroom scenes. She was also in my English class at school, and I thought she looked much nicer in rehearsal. Or maybe she just looked more tired and therefore more relaxed and open. But there was something about the music we moved to in the play, and about the awareness of attraction that Mildred's shenanigans were provoking, which combined to waken fresh feelings in me.

I may have wanted to be home rather than at rehearsal in the synagogue basement, but things there were growing more compelling. Soon Jacqueline began showing up in my dreams. So did Mildred, in varying states of dishevelment. It was as though her appearances as a man had intensified my sense of her as a woman, which in turn had ignited my interest in Jacqueline, who in turn was smiling at me in school.

When Oscar Hammerstein wrote to his friend Joshua Logan, who had directed the film version of *South Pacific*, that *The King and I* "is a very strange play and must be accepted on its own terms," he was thinking about its groundbreaking shortage of comedy and lack of traditional love story, its exotic historical setting and unfamiliar musical underpinnings, its hero's death at the end. He didn't have in mind the King being played by an actress in drag, who awakens an adolescent to feelings for his royal half sister.

The result of this deception is very strange to tell

The King and I is a work whose inspiration and narrative origins are rooted in transfiguration, trickery, misdirection, deceit, artful poses. The musical is, according to its official source credit, based on Margaret Landon's 1944 novel, *Anna and the King of Siam*. But when Rodgers and Hammerstein read the loosely plotted book, they weren't sure it had a strong enough story. Then they saw the 1946 movie adaptation, also called *Anna and the King of Siam*, which starred Rex Harrison and Irene Dunne, and was written by Sally Benson and Talbot Jennings. Afterward, writes Frederick Nolan in *The Sound of Their Music*, "Dick and Oscar knew at once it was a perfect vehicle for a musical." The movie offered a narrative line lacking in Landon's novel and developed an explicit attraction between Anna and the King, making him more charming. It provided him with an eccentric way of speaking, enriched minor characters, and introduced a subplot of the doomed young lovers Tuptim and Lun Tha.

But Landon's novel, despite her prefatory claim that it was "seventy-five per cent fact, and twenty-five percent fiction based on fact," was based upon two almost wholly fabricated memoirs written by Anna Leonowens, *The English Governess at the Siamese Court* (1870) and *The Romance of the Harem* (1872). Those memoirs, as exhaustively demonstrated in Susan Morgan's 2008 book, *Bombay Anna: The Real Story and Remarkable Adventures of the "King and I" Governess*, were "preposterous," an "invention." Morgan writes of Anna's arrival in the Far East: "At the moment Anna Leonowens disembarked, she reinvented herself. She simply made up a new 'history' of her origins and identity, a new biography." Morgan hits the point hard: "Anna was not an English lady. She was a fake."

The real Anna had been born in India, not Wales, in 1831 rather than 1834. She was the child of a young Anglo Indian widow and a deceased English soldier rather than of fully British parents, one of whom was a noble major. Her father died of illness, not in heroic combat, as Anna stated, "cut to pieces by Sikhs who lay in wait for him." Coming from a background of poverty and illiteracy, she "metamorphosed into the highly literate and polylingual Anna," and her "fantasy autobiography" is little more than "a charmingly romantic story, complete with a shipwreck and rescue, all aimed at establishing her and her children's racial and social claims to being British, white, and upper class." In addition, little of what Anna reports about her five years in Bangkok withstands historical scrutiny. Her summary of Siamese history, biographical sketch of Mongkut, presentation of life in the country, and portraits of its inhabitants are profoundly inaccurate.

So the enduring musical about a woman transformed by her experience in Bangkok, and transforming the world of Siam on the strength of her character and grit, is based on a movie based on a novel based on a memoir based on lies and falsehoods. Its heroine, so rigorous in defense of her authenticity and honesty, was in actuality a wizard of inauthenticity and dishonesty. Her character may have been strong, but not in the righteous way portrayed. Rather, it was strong enough to sustain an outlandish fraudulence.

Since the lyricist Oscar Hammerstein wouldn't have known about Anna's true backstory, it's ironic and prescient that Anna's first song is all about deception. Cheery, charming, "I Whistle a Happy Tune" concerns Anna's habit of pretending a calmness she doesn't feel, of whistling to cover up her fears:

> The result of this deception
> Is very strange to tell
> For when I fool the people
> I fear I fool myself as well!

Eerily, given the real-life Anna Leonowens's practices, the musical's Anna closes the song by urging her son to follow a similar course. She's passing along the legacy of deception as a social tool.

Hammerstein, who also wrote the play's dialogue, included numerous scenes in which Anna uses deception. She colludes with the young lovers, abetting their escape from the palace and Tuptim's liberation from the King's harem. She stages an elaborate dinner for visiting British dignitaries—with all the trappings of Western manners, behavior, customs of dress, and modes of dining, none of which are in fact customary within the palace—in order to suggest the King's European civility and to cover up what she knows to be his barbarity. She teaches the children songs and proverbs about the importance of a home, using her lessons as a means to remind their father of his broken promise to provide her with an independent apartment rather than a space in the palace. Her songs routinely celebrate various acts of subterfuge, not only whistling a happy tune to deceive yourself and others, but in "Hello, Young Lovers," when "you fly down a street on the chance that you meet, / and you meet— not really by chance," or in "Shall We Dance?," when a man and woman "say goodnight but mean goodbye."

Transformations, ruses, secrets, schemes, an overall mood of foxy cunning dominate the entire play. You're never sure who's being straightforward or honest. When we first meet the Kralahome—the King's prime minister—he pretends not to understand English, duping the newly arrived Anna into revealing too much about her thoughts and judgments as she speaks openly to her son and acquaintances. Called upon to advise the King in matters of diplomacy, Anna gains acceptance only by fooling him into believing her ideas to be his own. Lovers meet clandestinely, hiding from the moonlight. In one of its most memorable scenes, a dinnertime entertainment is presented to the British guests in which Harriet Beecher Stowe's *Uncle Tom's Cabin* is transformed into "The Small House of Uncle Thomas," a Siamese ballet replete with masks and jeweled headdresses and a buddha who changes a silk scarf into a frozen river. A celebration of Siamese culture and civility is turned into a critique of its barbaric practice of slavery.

Much of the music written for *The King and I* was composed to disguise its star's limitations as a singer. It was the first Rodgers and Hammerstein musical written for a specific performer, Gertrude Lawrence, who played Anna. According to Rodgers's autobiography, *Musical Stages*, Lawrence's lawyer brought Margaret Landon's novel to the composer's attention and "we were concerned that such an arrangement might not give us the freedom to write what we wanted the way we wanted." Despite this, they went ahead, further troubled by the fact that, as Rodgers knew, Lawrence was a poor singer. "We felt that her vocal range was minimal and that she had never been able to overcome an unfortunate tendency to sing flat." So Rodgers wrote songs for her "that were of relatively limited range while saving the more demanding arias and duets for those singers whose voices could handle them."

Then, in a play designed for Lawrence, and with her appearing as both star and central point of view, they wrote a part for the King and cast the charismatic, versatile Yul Brynner, transforming the play into a vehicle for him instead. Brynner became so identified with the role, performing it on stage nearly five thousand times, winning the leading actor Tony Award, then winning the best actor Oscar in the 1956 film version, and even starring in a short-lived 1972 television series called *Anna and the King*, that he hijacked a show in which his role was conceived as secondary. As Ethan Mordden notes in *Coming Up Roses*, his 1998 book about the Broadway musical in the 1950s, "Yul Brynner began to crowd the Annas, and, in two major revivals, it was he who got solo headline billing."

Something wonderful

In our community theater production, my mother played Lady Thiang, the King's head wife, described in the novel as "the most important of the royal wives." It was in many respects a dream-come-true for her, because my mother adored the notion of being royalty, even if only through pretense, and she felt quite comfortable being the most important royal woman around. I remember her telling friends *of course I'm really almost the Queen*, and queenly is how she portrayed the character. It was unjust, my mother said, that the program didn't bill her, along with Mildred and Blanche—the woman who played Anna—among the show's stars.

The role required my mother to perform one operatic piece, "Something Wonderful." Sung directly to Anna, it's crucial to the plot, allowing Lady Thiang to reveal why she loves the difficult, capricious King, despite his many flaws. "This is a man who thinks with his heart, / His heart is not always wise," she explains to Anna. Few of his dreams will be realized, but at least he has dreams and believes in them. The King needs love, is capable of giving love, and if loved "he'll do something wonderful." These insights soften Anna's view of him and convince her, at least temporarily, of the King's humanity and the worthiness of her own role in his kingdom.

"Something Wonderful" is a tough song to perform. As Thomas Hischak notes in *The Oxford Companion to the American Musical*, it "has a direct and unfussy lyric while Rodgers' music soars with emotion." So its delivery requires both technical precision and a deep clarity of feeling. The song works best if the singer underplays, trusting the power of Rodgers's music. It was one of those "demanding arias" Rodgers mentioned, "written for a singer whose voice could handle them," and it presented my mother with a serious challenge. She had good vocal chops, had performed on radio and in the 1930s and in our home for friends, but years of Chesterfields had lowered and coarsened her voice and had combined with extra weight and lack of exercise to limit her breathing capacity. I didn't know what kind of singer she'd been in her heyday, but for as long as I'd been hearing her, she used song as a means of self-display. Playing for friends in our living room, she would bat her eyes and roll her head, pound on the piano, stand abruptly, and flop back down onto her bench. I was prepared to be embarrassed by her Lady Thiang. But her performance was impressive, and though she had to talk-sing much of "Something Wonderful," that only made more powerful the moments when she let her voice soar. Having imagined her winking, wiggling her hips, and overemoting, I was astounded by her command.

I was also muddled by the premise behind the song and its delivery. My mother was being moved to such unprecedented grandeur by her feelings for Mildred Levine? Sure, it was a transmogrified Mildred Levine, but still, I was having trouble seeing past the artifice.

And look what Mildred as the King had done to my mother as his wife: married her, shunted her aside for twenty-two other wives, favored the children of other wives, and yet inspired her to maintain this tenacious love. Where was that loyal, loving, forgiving, self-contained version of my mother when we were all at home, where my mother was so angry, volatile, and bitter?

I couldn't help wondering about that because, when wearing her bald headpiece, Mildred brought to mind my father. Sometimes I imagined my mother was singing "Something Wonderful" about him, though she always made it clear that she thought he was the most un-wonderful and undeserving man among the hundreds who had courted her. The Greatest Mistake of Her Life.

While we were rehearsing and performing *The King and I* in our synagogue on Long Island, my wheelchair-bound father was living five nights a week in a New York City apartment with my brother, having spent the previous two years recovering from injuries sustained in a car wreck. With my brother's support, he was able to return to work as a factory foreman in Manhattan's garment district, but commuting two hours a day was impossible. So they came home on weekends, exhausted, and the whole way of life in our family—in the Skloot Kingdom—remained in flux. My father, the diminished leader, seemed nearly powerless, confined, dependent, and my mother was now cavorting with a new and strange leader, Monday through Friday, greeting my father's weekend returns as a burden, an interruption of her more real life in the theater.

I tried not to resent him for putting me in the situation of bit player in *The King and I* and in my mother's theatrical life. But because my father and brother were gone all week and my mother was going to be at rehearsals, and because my parents were unwilling to let me be at home by myself those evenings, I was forced to participate in the show. I had one line to speak during a classroom scene ("What is that green over there?"), one line to sing solo in "Getting to Know You" ("Suddenly I'm bright and breezy"), and a formal bow to master in "The March of the Siamese Children." For that, I had to be at rehearsal every night, not at home alone where I promised to do all my homework and three extra-credit reports per week, where I could watch *Surfside Six* or *The Rifleman, Rawhide,* or *Hawaiian Eye.* Or where, as my teenage years began, I could explore feelings connected with seeing Tuesday Weld as Thalia Menninger on *The Many Loves of Dobie Gillis* rather than dealing with Mildred Levine in her various manifestations. Well, at least there was Jacqueline, who did look a little like Tuesday Weld.

To this day, more than fifty years after *The King and I* finished its two-night run, I remember all the lyrics to all the songs and can speak most of the dialogue along with the actors on stage or screen. In 1998, when Beverly and I saw Maureen McGovern's traveling production in Portland, I wept and whispered my way through it despite the glares from those sitting nearby.

When he has looked at me what has he seen?

Tuptim, the young woman transported from Burma and given as a gift to the King, voices one of the play's central themes when she sings "My Lord and Master." This is a song whose lyrics are completely open about the subject of hiddenness, speaking directly about the gulf between a character's appearance and reality. Because the King has told her so, Tuptim knows he's pleased with her. But, she asks, "What does he mean? / What does he know of me?" What pleases him are her youthful looks, smile, and shining eyes, which he assumes to be shining solely for him. These appealing visible signs make Tuptim an acceptable addition to the King's collection of wives. But she's withholding her essential self, the part she has given in love to Lun Tha. And though the King may study her as hard as he can,

"The smile beneath my smile / He'll never see." She has masked her true persona and offered him a conventional, formal image instead. "When he has looked at me what has he seen?" Hurt, sad, abused, Tuptim nevertheless sings a delicate, yearning melody, all the more powerful for its tenderness and poise.

Ironically, given its roots tangled in inauthenticity and false identity, and its many instances of fraudulence, *The King and I* is about maintaining an authentic and truthful identity, about knowing and being true to yourself, especially during times of great personal and societal change. It's concerned with the integrity of the self when that integrity is threatened.

Anna, newly widowed, newly relocated to a strange and alien culture, is under intense pressure. She's lonely and grieving, far from home and familiar ways, challenged to instruct the King's children while also looking out for her son's best interests, which may not always coincide with the royal family's. She's overwhelmed by feelings for her students, for their mothers within the harem, and eventually for the King himself, for whom she feels both attraction and repulsion. He places mercurial and sometimes humiliating demands on her, demands that seem aimed at shattering her pretensions: she's ordered to grovel like a toad, her head kept in a lower position than his own even when he's lying on the floor; she must live in his palace rather than in the independent apartment agreed to by contract; she must acknowledge herself as his slave; she's ordered to be a diplomatic advisor in addition to schoolteacher. These threaten Anna's sense of independence, authority, and purpose, and she nearly loses herself in the swarm of commands, responsibilities, and conflicts. At the beginning, she can distract herself from it all, whistling her tune. But eventually the threat to her identity is too serious for such remedies, and her musical soliloquies become cluttered with confusion, contradiction, and the feeling that she must leave Siam—with nowhere else to go—before it destroys everything she believes about herself.

The aging King rules at a time of cultural upheaval as his country, exposed to modernization and foreign influence, threatened by British colonial expansion, drifts away from the certainties that sustained his power. And Anna, whom he has invited into his sanctum, only deepens the threat even as she gains his trust. As Meryle Secrest notes in *Somewhere for Me*, her biography of Richard Rodgers, the King is "a man at the crossroads: inheritor of a feudal tradition who takes his godlike status for granted, yet cannot help being thrown into doubt by the challenge to his set of values that his European schoolmistress represents." It's a time when the absolutes that supported his core beliefs are no longer credible. He expresses the dilemma in his great solo number, "A Puzzlement," about the difference between his simple understanding of the world when he was a boy and the more nuanced understanding he has as King:

> Now I am a man;
> World have changed a lot:
> Some things nearly so,
> Others nearly not.

The drama being played out by both main characters is one of honest presentation of self. How can each remain true to that self when it is no longer stable? When outside circumstances shift the very basis of self-knowledge? This drama is echoed by the issues affecting other characters as well: the spurned royal wife sustaining herself by love and pride; the young lovers forced apart by an arranged marriage to the King; the Kralahome, resistant to change but recognizing its necessity. All must figure out how to act with integrity, how to change without losing touch with who they are.

Here at the onset of my teen years, when the chief struggle was to make identity coalesce and stabilize, and then to find an honest presentation of self, I was for two intense months immersed in the inauthentic. Looking back across the five decades, I see that those months were important in shaping my sense of what love might be.

There was, of course, the music, particularly the haunting, hopeful love songs that give *The King and I* a quality Ethan Mordden calls "tragic rhapsody." I was particularly drawn to the young lovers' two passionate songs, "I Have Dreamed" and "We Kiss in a Shadow." Both celebrate the power of romantic and erotic imagination, something I was just beginning to appreciate myself.

Lun Tha opens "I Have Dreamed" by revealing that he has pictured himself in Tuptim's embrace, has fantasized in ways that even 1950s euphemisms can't obscure: "I have dreamed that your arms are lovely, / I have dreamed what a joy you'll be." He has imagined her intimate voice ("every word you whisper") and, indeed, feels sure he knows and will enjoy how it will feel to be loved by her. I was pretty sure I understood what he was singing about. And then Tuptim sings the same things back to him. What a revelation that was for me: girls have the same thoughts! Even now, in 2012 and after hearing the songs hundreds of times, when both lovers sing together in the song's final moment, saying they will love being loved by each other, I feel genuine sensual joy. Imagining love liberated from constraint is at the heart of "We Kiss in a Shadow," too. The clandestine lovers, unable to express their passion openly, long for freedom:

> To kiss in the sunlight
> And say to the sky:
> Behold and believe what you see!
> Behold how my lover loves me!

Seeing it, singing it, emerges in this scene as a convincing act of love. I found their songs, despite the tragic outcome of their story, to be almost unbearably stimulating.

When Anna sings "Hello, Young Lovers," giving Tuptim and Lun Tha her blessing, the mixture of longing and desire and passion for a connection that isn't available to her always stirs me. In many ways, the central lines of her song shaped my expectations for love: "I know how it feels to have wings on your heels, / And to fly down the street in a trance." I remain, at sixty-five, a wings-on-your-heels, fly-down-the-street romantic, as Beverly can attest. Someone moved to tears by the combination of song and physicality that made "Shall We Dance?" sexy, even when sung by a polka-spinning Mildred and Blanche in the synagogue auditorium.

For me, the love songs held out hope, and affirmed that it was okay to imagine and want the sort of romantic love given life in the musical. They provided me with notions—however skewed—of what might be possible beyond what I'd witnessed or experienced in my life. My parents' way wasn't the only way. I think the songs helped me form an ideal of love that involved tenderness, reciprocity, responsiveness, expressiveness, a meeting of mutually open and honest selves. Love in sharp contrast to all the deception, secrecy, posturing, and pretension in and around *The King and I*.

In addition to the music, there were also the love stories embodied in the play. As Meryle Secrest says, "*The King and I* is really a celebration of love in all its guises, from the love of Anna for her dead husband; the love of the King's official wife, Lady Thiang, for a man she knows is flawed and also unfaithful; the desperation of forbidden love; and a love that is barely recognized and can never be acted upon." Love was all around, almost all of it hidden, thwarted, subverted.

A bright cloud of music

My mother contributed more than her acting and singing talent. She also helped with costumes, designing elaborate crowns for the King and Prince and a rhinestone-studded sash for Lady Thiang to wear while singing "Something Wonderful." She made a crown for herself as well, worn only around the house to help her perfect Lady Thiang's regal character and bearing. She fabricated lavish ornaments to be used on the royal table during the big dinner scene. A few nights, she substituted for the regular pianist during rehearsals. After the play closed, my mother occasionally spoke in her character's pidgin English, unable to let go fully of her royal experience. The hauteur, the aristocratic bearing and expectation, the authority appealed to her sense of who she really was and how the world should see her.

And within eighteen months, she would—like Lady Thiang at the play's end—need to inhabit the role of widow. My father died suddenly at fifty-three, in a hotel swimming pool, during a Veterans Day vacation with my mother. Not long afterward, and with the score of *The King and I* still stuck in my head, I remember walking on the beach and hearing snatches of its songs as though they were carried on the breakers. One line in particular kept coming back, rolling over itself like a wave: *On a bright cloud of music shall we fly?* Walking home again, I also remembered a line that Anna speaks to her son during the play's *finale ultimo* as the King lies dying. Louis asks her if she and the King are friends again and Anna replies, "I suppose so, Louis. We can't hurt each other anymore." This seemed so apropos of my parents that it brought a kind of release for me, a glimpse of other ways to think about loss. Clearly, I was having a hard time letting go of *The King and I* too.

Jacqueline was my girlfriend at the time of my father's death. She wore the ring I'd been given to celebrate my bar mitzvah, which had taken place at the same synagogue where *The King and I* was performed. For months before I gave her the ring, we'd meet after school and walk home rather than ride the school bus. We talked, and I discovered that she was so pale and tired looking because she had a problem in her heart, and that she wanted to live in a big city rather than on an island, and that she wanted to be a kind of doctor I hadn't heard about, one who listens to people talk about their problems.

She was the first person I ever told about the way my parents behaved inside our home, the rages, the violence. One afternoon, having walked her home and then started toward my own, closer to the beach, I saw sunlight wink off the water and stopped, thinking that I really felt comfortable being myself with Jacqueline, and that I needed a moment to become the guarded, watchful person I was at home. And I began to whistle a tune from *The King and I*.

Shortly after my father's funeral, during the seven-day period of mourning known as sitting shivah, I remember a visit from Mildred Levine. She came to our house along with her husband, Vance, and my friend Richard, dressed in black, wearing her crimson lipstick and her blonde hair piled on top of her head, looking glamorous. Our living room was like a stage set, with hard benches for the immediate family to sit on throughout the week, all the mirrors covered in cloth, none of the men in the family shaving, each of us wearing torn black ribbons on our chests. Near the fireplace a table loaded with food looked like the table in the play's banquet scene. After expressing her condolences and sharing a few memories of my father, Mildred told us that she and her family were moving to California. She was going to try her luck in Hollywood. It took a while, but six years later, now known as Millie Levin, she appeared on television in two episodes of *Bewitched*, playing a secretary. A female secretary.

2

SENIOR SPEECH

I usta tawk like dis. Worse, really. *Woise.* Because I was born in Brooklyn, then moved at age ten to Long Beach, a small barrier island off the south shore of Long Island. *Lawn Guylin.* So I grew up speaking with a New Yorky hybrid of two heavy, distinctive, widely ridiculed American accents: Brooklynese, which is spoken through the gut, and Lawn Guylinese, which is spoken through the nose. Yeah, no less an authority than the BBC says Americans judge these particular accents to be "the most unpleasant and most incorrect" in the entire United States. What's more, even those who speak them "don't really like their accents either." And according to the linguistics scholar William Labov, in his book *The Social Stratification of English in New York City*, "as far as language is concerned, New York City may be characterized as a sink of negative prestige." *Dat hoits!*

It's culturally tainted speech. Not just pronunciation, but the entire delivery system—tone, cadence, rhythm, inflection, attitude, speed, articulation—is implicated. People hear the accent, hear you say *I p'fuh Wawluss Shtevens's oily voice* when you mean you prefer Wallace Stevens's early verse, and they make negative judgments about your intelligence, character, class. About your level of couth, even if you can recite the first lines of Stevens's "Sunday Morning" by heart, saying *Kimplaysunzees udda pinwah, an late / Cawfee n'arnjizz inna sunny cheahr* instead of "Complacencies of the peignoir, and late / Coffee and oranges in a sunny chair."

The *Wall Street Journal* reports that if you "exhibit an abrasive Brooklyn accent, you risk derailing your career because you appear unpolished." Actors with staunch New York accents end up playing gangsters, hard hats, punch-drunk boxers, cops, bartenders. It's a hard, grimy, pounded sound, a street-sound that in 1946 led Edmund Wilson, in *Memoirs of Hecate County*, to express his disdain by calling it "an accent worn down on the lips of the crowd as the long Brooklyn pavements had been by their feet." Mashed, raggedy, tattered, low. In the 1993 movie *Life with Mikey*, a character mocked for calling Sunburst cookies *Sunboist cookies* responds by saying, "Hey, I'm from Brooklyn, you're lucky I can speak English."

C'mon, fuggedaboutit!

My father, a chicken butcher born and raised in Brooklyn, called the toilet *duh terlet*. He usually called me *Flerd* instead of Floyd and said that the infielder Billy Cox of the Dodgers played *toid* rather than third. When our food was cooked in olive *earl*, it was good enough to serve to the *Dook uv Oil*. That phonetic reversal of *oy* and *er*—the upgliding central diphthong that turns *curl* to *coil* and *coil* to *curl*—invites derision, as William Labov notes: its "use in any context is now heavily stigmatized." Labov also says that "on radio and television, stereotypes of middle-class and working-class New York City speech have traditionally been used for comic effects." No wonder he found that "the term 'linguistic self-hatred' is not too extreme to apply to the situation."

A serious teenaged boy, desperate to be considered suave and polished and well read, I didn't need to provoke mirth on the basis of my accent. But I sounded coarse. My father (and then I) had the full array of stigmatized quirks in addition to the upgliding central diphthong. We had the dropped *h* and *r*, the dropped *t* and *g*, that made people like us say *I tawt you wuh goin wit me, young fella.* We had the trifecta of *dem, deez,* and *doze*; substituted *aks* for *ask*; turned *pork* into *pawk.* If my father didn't like the way I looked, he'd ask *whut's amattah witchoo?* To which I would reply *nuttin.* Fed up, he'd say, *ahhh, g'wahn* or *yuh faddah's moostash,* and flick his hand at me. *I'm tellinya duh troot heeah.*

These were all regular elements of our household speech, along with the intensity, emphasis, volume, and gesture that made it seem as if we were always arguing, always jabbing our fingers in people's faces. Pugnacious, edgy, volatile. My parents were, in fact, pugnacious, edgy, volatile. Between themselves, and with their two sons, they were brutally explosive, filled with fury, and because of their accents they sounded dangerous even when they weren't. There was this consistency between my parents' action and manner of expression that has long darkened my sense of New York speech and still makes me tense when I hear it anywhere.

§

It wasn't my father's fault that he sounded the way he did. He came by his accent almost as naturally as he'd come by his lack of height and hair, or the butcher's trade his parents and older brother also shared. His father, who left the village of Volozhin in Russia's Pale of Settlement at the age of twelve, in 1892, had died a decade before I was born, so I never heard him speak except in the voices of his six children. They all sounded like my father, even the sisters who married wealthy, upper-class men. And as I remember, my father's mother, from Bialystok in eastern Poland, often didn't use words at all. She spoke with eloquent sighs and grunts and moans, all of which had accents. The depth of her dismay was easily determined by the duration and pitch of her *oyyyyyych*, her *hmmmmmmm*, her *phphphphphhhhh*. It was speech reduced to pure inflection, and I would sometimes hear sounds like hers in certain kosher delicatessens or in my father's poultry market. Though he'd finished high school, gone on to own a live poultry market, was considered a sharp and savvy guy, my father retained the accent of his kin and clan, and his boyhood was no breeding ground for the proper enunciation of Standard American English.

But of course there was more than my Brooklyn father and neighborhood influences contributing to my accent. My mother, who left school after the ninth grade, was the daughter of more expressive, more outgoing eastern European Jewish immigrants. They were furriers with an uptown clientele, and their densely accented English, seasoned with Yiddish and topped with Polish, seemed chewed rather than spoken. They talked animatedly, waving their hands, my grandfather struggling to keep his false teeth from popping out as he carried on conversation. He would hear horns honking on the New York City street below his apartment window and say *I kin told difference from boss and tsixie-kep jist fum de sound horn* when he meant that he can tell the difference between a bus and taxicab just from hearing the sounds of their horns. He would order me to *dill de cotts* instead of deal the cards when we played *chin rommy*. My grandmother would call me *Floit* as she *zoived de zoop* which she admitted was *vundafel* and my grandfather said was *werry gutt*.

They sounded like the speech-challenged adult students preparing for naturalization exams, the source of so much humor in Leo Rosten's 1937 novel, *The Education of H*Y*M*A*N K*A*P*L*A*N*, in which the title character speaks of George Washington "fightink for Friddom, against the Kink of Ingland, Kink Jawdge Number Tree, dat tarrible autocrap."

My mother grew up amid these accents while living in the Bronx and then Manhattan. She aspired to stardom as a singer-actress on stage and radio, aspired to aristocracy in marriage, and eventually claimed both stardom and aristocracy when they were denied her. To support this claim, she concocted a wildly theatrical accent that combined those of movie stars she considered royalty, such as Zsa Zsa Gabor or Marlene Dietrich, with those of French chanteuses, Russian ballerinas, and imaginary Romanian countesses, adding occasional Britishisms adopted from her cousin-by-marriage, Jean Alfus. All shot through with New York and Yiddish overtones. I can still remember her gasping when she saw a dirty vase in our living room, putting a hand over her bosom, and saying *oy dahlink, that goooorjus vaaaahze is so doidy*.

ⓢ

I didn't stand a phonetic chance. According to British linguist David Crystal in *By Hook or by Crook*, accents "get established very early in life. Children have them by the age of three." *Ay muddah, I gotta go to duh bat'trum*. And though it may be true, as psychologist Steven Pinker says in *The Language Instinct*, that "children of immigrants always grow up with the accents of their peers, not those of their parents," my mother and father had heavily accented peers in their New York backgrounds. So did I. Where we came from, and who we hung out with, remained essentially working-class Jewish people. Our way of talking didn't really move toward conformity with middle-class norms of speech because we were seldom among people who spoke it. This was true during our Brooklyn years, when we lived in a large apartment building and socialized primarily with family, neighbors in the building, and a few people from the local synagogue or my father's world of butchers, bakers, longshoremen. It was also true during our Long Beach years, both before and after my father's death in 1961, when most of our friends and neighbors were themselves recent working-class transplants from Brooklyn, Queens, the Bronx, or Manhattan.

Once we relocated, my speech added some Long Islandisms to the already bizarre blend: the doubled vowel that turns *hat* into *hay-at*, the drawling *aw* that turns a *mall* into a two-syllable *mawull* or *wash* into *warsh*, the added *h* that turns Skloot into *Shkloot*, the gulped *er* that turns *her* into *huh*. Right, the dapper young man *warshed up, den waugh a hayut to meet huh at de mawull.*

This all made for a presentation of my teenage self that was raw rather than refined, much rougher than the smooth guy I hoped to project. I was Archie Bunker. I was Ralph Kramden with a little bit of Joey Buttafuoco thrown in. I was freakin' Bugs Bunny, the Jewish version. Yet I wanted so earnestly to separate myself from the environment in which I was raised. I wanted to assert my difference from parents who screamed and fought, angry all the time, who hit their children, never read books, traveled no farther from New York than Connecticut. I was obsessed with being unlike them, being my own self, growing more sophisticated and worldly, getting away from my family. But I sure sounded like I belonged right there with them.

ṣ

George Bernard Shaw's 1914 play, *Pygmalion*, is about the London phonetician Henry Higgins, who teaches a tattered flower-seller named Eliza Doolittle to lose her Cockney accent, thereby calling forth her inner Lady, transforming her character and life. Transformed itself into the 1956 Broadway musical *My Fair Lady*, where "The Rain in Spain" turns an elocution lesson into a memorable song, *Pygmalion* focuses on the liberating power of accent-free, standardized speech. Also of manners and dress, but the main point is that proper speech is the key to overcoming socioeconomic, class, or cultural obstacles to success and self-realization. Without her Cockney accent and ways, Eliza is able to pass as a duchess at a high-society ball. Change speech and you not only change destiny, open up opportunities, but you change something vital inside as well. Metamorphosis through correct diction.

In the play's preface, Shaw writes, "For the encouragement of people troubled with accents that cut them off from all high employment, I may add that the change wrought by Professor Higgins in the flower girl is neither impossible nor uncommon." But, he warns, "the thing has to be done scientifically, or the last state of the aspirant may be worse than the first."

When I was seventeen, it was Mrs. Selma Sherman who did the thing scientifically to me and to about two dozen other members of the Long Beach High School senior speech class in 1964–65. I'd been hearing about senior speech and Mrs. Sherman for two years, since moving up from junior high, though I'd never met her in person. She was voted "Favorite Teacher" every year. According to *Echo*, the high school yearbook, senior speech was "one of the most popular courses" and "an important pre-college preparation." It was also supposed to be easy, at least in terms of workload, just a few speeches to prepare and deliver. All good reasons to sign up, but my attention was really caught by the course description: "It is vital to speak well for what you believe. On this basis, Mrs. Sherman guides her senior classes toward a mode of speech that will gain respect for them in the future." Speaking well, gaining respect; my main motivation for enrolling was an increasing sense of urgency about sounding different, sounding right.

At fifteen, I'd auditioned for a summer camp production of *West Side Story* and was cast as A-Rab, one of the Jets. At our first read-through, the director gathered her Jets stage right and said she'd cast each of us because, of all who'd tried out and could sing and dance, we sounded the most like kids who could be in a New York street gang. Our accents were perfect for hoodlums. "Doan get fancy on me, awright? Just tawk duh way you tawk."

Her remark, and the way she continued to harp on our diction, made me hyperaware of how I sounded, with all that implied. And I began to pay attention to speech. Well, sometimes I paid attention, but the only model I had for correction was the cockamamie medley of accents in my mother's repertoire. So I would say things like *I doan wanna loin howta dahhnce*. As George Bernard Shaw had warned those lacking a scientific approach, this particular aspirant's state was getting worse than before he tried to fix it. Clearly, I needed professional help.

I remember my first senior speech class vividly, nearly fifty years after it met. In her yearbook photograph, Mrs. Sherman had looked a bit bobbed and Betty Crockerish, with short hair waved high in front like a pompadour and carefully curled at the sides. Very 1950s. So the first surprise was how elegant and *au courant* she appeared, dressed in a dark V-neck outfit, white piping at the neck and pockets, her black hair in a top-heavy mop. She stood in front of her desk and leaned comfortably back against it, smiling at us. Closer than if she were behind the desk, but still formal and very much in control of the room, just by her glance. When she spoke, she sounded exactly like what she was: a former dramatic arts major at New York University, with some television and radio work in her background.

I felt immediately relaxed as she told us about the four or five speeches we would give and about the sounds she wanted us to become aware of. *The man can have an apple.* She scanned the room, smiled, then found me and stopped everything.

"Stand up," Mrs. Sherman said. Then she asked my name and nodded when she found it in her gradebook. "Get rid of your gum, Mr. Skloot." I had been chewing my Juicy Fruit with such minimal jaw movements that I was astounded to be caught. As I walked toward the garbage can, she spoke to the class. "Gum chewing marks you every bit as much as an accent does."

It's difficult to hear your own accent. Most of us are seldom conscious of our voices as we speak, of pronunciation, the actual sound of language. That's why it's so shocking to hear our recorded voices on the telephone answering machine or on radio. We're usually not aware of our facial expressions or gestures either, the sorts of character-defining communication business that actors pay attention to. We just talk.

Until we're forced to stop and listen. Brenda Maddox, the Massachusetts-born biographer of James Joyce's wife, Nora, William Butler Yeats and his wife, Georgie, and D.H. Lawrence and his wife, Frieda, has devoted most of her professional life to the subject of intimate communications. Married to the physicist and science writer Sir John Maddox, she has lived in London since the early 1960s and, fed up with being mistaken for a tourist and wanting to feel more deeply connected to her community, she actively sought to lose her American accent. In a 1999 article about that experience for the *New Statesman*, Maddox says that after hiring a voice coach, her greatest challenge was learning to hear properly. "Quite soon I learnt that I had been deaf all these years. I thought I was adapting to native speech simply by saying 'GARage' instead of 'garAGE' and 'tewlips' instead of 'toolips.'" Unlike Eliza Doolittle in *Pygmalion*, Maddox never does fool the locals or shed her outsiderness, though her own family back in Massachusetts "thinks I sound like the Queen." Perhaps she lacks the essential criterion noted by Professor Higgins, who says he can help Eliza lose her accent quickly only "if she has a good ear."

The New York "accent reduction" teacher Alan Kennedy, interviewed for a Columbia University News Service article, confirms the necessity for a good ear. "The first step," Kennedy says, "is to help students hear the English words they're saying that sound un-American." He's referring to students of English as a second language. But it makes sense to me that the same you-have-to-hear-it-first principle would apply to heavily accented native English speakers, whose accents can deviate from the norm nearly as much as a foreigner's does. If Standard American English—the sound of the Great American Nowhere, the accentless speech of network news broadcasters—is that norm, then the sound pattern of my childhood New York speech was pretty close to a foreign accent. *Wud'nit?*

When Mrs. Sherman's class began in 1964, I was already conscious of the way I sounded, was motivated to change, and had a good enough ear that I could mimic my grandparents' accents, get a laugh with my Irish brogue, imitate a Russian spymaster, and had sung my portion of "Gee, Officer Krupke" in *West Side Story* using the German accent required by the script. But I hadn't put together the notion that such mimicry might be a key to clearing up my accent. And I still lacked a steady model to mimic.

"Feel your mouth work," Mrs. Sherman told us. *The cat sat on a ramp and ate carrots.* "Look at the person sitting next to you, watch the mouth." *Rownd.* "Break it down: ahh-ooo equals the sound in *round.*"

More than mimicry was involved, though. Because at age seventeen, learning to speak differently was like learning a foreign language. We were coming to the challenge a little late in our development. Young children pick up second languages, including appropriate accents, with astonishing facility. But, as Steven Pinker says, it's hard for most adults to master a foreign language, and the phonology is especially hard because speech development "often fossilizes into permanent error patterns." The key factor in learning to speak a new language properly is a person's age. "People who immigrate after puberty provide some of the most compelling examples." Pinker cites Henry Kissinger, who came to America as a teenager, learned English grammar very well, but still speaks with a heavy German accent. His younger brother, however, has no accent. Vladimir Nabokov is a similar example, a late arrival to English who became a brilliant stylist of the written language but spoke with a strong Russian accent. Pinker notes Nabokov's own assessment: "I write like a distinguished author, and I speak like a child."

As late teens, our speech pattern as we entered Mrs. Sherman's class was already hardwired in our brains, so the accent-cleansing process had a significant neurological component. We needed to reprogram speech centers having entrenched neurochemical pathways. Eliza Doolittle says learning to speak properly "was just like learning to dance in the fashionable way." Others have compared it to changing eating habits to lose weight and keep it off, or learning to hit a baseball when all you've played since your teenage years was basketball, or mastering martial arts at middle age. What these comparisons all suggest is that changing an accent is very much a physical activity as well as a mental one. The effort is to make the new way become second nature. It requires concentration and repetition, and it isn't easy. We've all seen our share of bad dancers / failed dieters / lousy hitters / awkward kung-fu practitioners.

Mrs. Sherman, using what linguist William Labov calls "the mechanism of imitation and hypercorrection," was seeking to unnewyork us. To pull a Professor Higgins on us. The movie version of *My Fair Lady* came out during the Christmas holiday of 1964 and reinforced what Mrs. Sherman was teaching. Maybe we wouldn't pass for dukes and duchesses, but we might be able to climb out of that sink of negative prestige.

ى

When Francie Nolan, the main character in Betty Smith's 1943 novel, *A Tree Grows in Brooklyn*, is thinking about attending Columbia University in Manhattan or Long Island's Adelphi University, both near home, a family friend says she should "go far off to college—she might get rid of her Brooklyn accent that way." But Francie is not so sure that's a good idea. She "didn't want to get rid of it any more than she wanted to get rid of her name" because "it meant that she *belonged* some place. She was a Brooklyn girl with a Brooklyn name and a Brooklyn accent. She didn't want to change into a bit of this and a bit of that."

Brooklyn-born folk singer Arlo Guthrie also resisted efforts to eradicate his accent. According to Arlo's sister, Nora, in Michael W. Robbins's *Brooklyn: A State of Mind*, their mother hired a British drama and speech teacher to correct their accents. She remembers her brothers "riding in the car on the Belt Parkway, saying 'Don't! Don't! Don't!' sometimes in a Brooklyn accent and sometimes not." Their father, Woody, spoke and sang with an Okie twang, and Arlo liked his own Brooklyn accent. "Even now, when you listen to Arlo's records, you can hear this accent," Nora says. "The way he pronounces the words is pure Brooklyn."

According to David Crystal, "accents exist to express your identity. They tell people where you are from." They "identify communities." As Crystal notes, Professor Higgins in *Pygmalion* claims that just by hearing someone speak he "can place a man within six miles" of his community. "Within two miles in London. Sometimes within two streets."

There's a flip side to the various sociological, economic, cultural arguments in favor of losing an accent. While Mrs. Sherman wished "to improve everybody's speech, so they sounded like well-educated people" and help us "gain respect," and while William Labov writes about "the pressures toward conformity with middle class norms of speech" and finds that New Yorkers "would be complimented if someone told them they did not sound like New Yorkers," there is Francie Nolan's legitimate desire to retain her accent and with it retain her sense of belonging, her sense of home. She connects her accent with a kind of integrity of being, and fears that moving away and losing her distinctive speech would begin a process of fragmentation, of "change into a bit of this and a bit of that." Arlo Guthrie, too, sought to retain his community link and, probably, to further separate his voice from his father's Okie sound. I suppose, too, that holding on to a strong accent like Francie's or Guthrie's, like mine, would have been a statement of allegiance to place and to the past, to origins.

But I wanted the opposite. Escape, that was my obsession. Disallegiance. I refused to attend nearby Hofstra University, where my mother wanted me to go, applying only to out-of-state schools, and bought in completely to Mrs. Sherman's philosophy. I believed that cleaned-up speech would liberate me. And I was beginning to grasp that sounding "normal" in *how* I said something might shift more attention onto *what* I said. I became a passionate convert.

We were assigned to give a five-minute speech that taught our classmates how to do something—paint a watercolor flower, shoot free throws, change a flat tire—about which we felt expert. I spoke about cooking a ham and cheese omelet, and, ever my mother's son, spent the last minute in a detailed account of the best technique for scouring the pan and stovetop afterward. We were required to sit across the desk from Mrs. Sherman, shake her hand, and undergo a practice college interview during which we were scored both for what we said and how we enunciated it. Assigned to give a speech about something that moved us, I spoke publicly, for the first time, about my father's death three years earlier, using as my prop a medal he'd won as a high school track star. I remember rushing back to my seat, face suffused with heat, refusing to look up, trying not to cry but also furious with myself because I knew the only serious mistake I'd made was with the speech's final word. *Fawddah.* I was, I think, becoming a seriously conscious speaker.

In the fall of 2008, I spent a month trying to find Selma Sherman again. Google was little help, especially since I couldn't remember her first name or decipher her signature in my yearbook. At the school district offices, no one knew who I was talking about, and said that if they had known, they wouldn't be able to give me information about her anyway. They did provide an e-mail address for the current principal of the high school, and I wrote to explain what I was looking for. He didn't reply, but a couple of weeks later I heard from Mrs. Sherman's daughter, Ronda, who wrote that her mother not only was alive and living in Florida, but was about to arrive in New York for a Thanksgiving family visit. Ronda, following her mother's footsteps, had taught at Long Beach High School for many years. She had also, a few years after me, taken her mother's senior speech class. Mrs. Sherman—Selma—was eighty-six, in good health, and would be glad to talk with me.

I loved interviewing her. She said she'd taught until 1975, ten years after I last saw her. She'd remarried and wanted to travel. Teaching had been something she got into accidentally, a job she took upon moving to Long Beach with her first husband in the mid-1950s. "I loved working with sixteen- to eighteen-year-olds," she said. "They were people already."

We were, and that made her task harder because our language habits had solidified. At the same time, the teenage years are about inventing or reinventing yourself, shaping an adult identity. It's a fluid period perfect for taking senior speech, when the goals of the course and the goals of the student—some of them, at least—are in harmony. Change speech and change destiny.

Near the end of our recent conversation, Selma said, "You know, Floyd, you speak without any trace of an accent now." It felt like the moment I got my real grade from her.

But I lapse sometimes. *Id'nat sump'n?* It happens when I talk to my daughter's boyfriend, David Prete, who's from Yonkers. He's a trained actor, having graduated from the New Actors Workshop in New York where he studied with Mike Nichols, and his New York accent has been scrubbed too. But together, we fall into our old speech patterns. *Hahya dooin?* when we see each other, or *Wairs duh sawlt?* when we're cooking together. At first, it's a joke, a performance. It's play. But then it starts to take hold, and I need to concentrate in order to sound like myself again. Or it happens when I'm in New York, especially in shops or restaurants and coffee shops, places where things start to get pushy and urgent. It also happens when I'm with my cousins, six or seven Skloots in a Manhattan living room cackling over Joe Pesci's Brooklyn accent in the 1992 movie *My Cousin Vinny*: *D'ja heah him sayin "deez yutes" steada "these youths"?* Sometimes, even here in laid-back Oregon, it happens when I drive in heavy traffic. *Ay! Watch whutcha dooin, joik-wad!* It even happens, for no discernible reason, maybe just a glitch of aging or failure of attention, as when I said to Beverly over dinner last night, *dis chicken tastes good, dud'nit?*

So my work on the accent is still in progress. Just writing this essay, never mind reading it aloud, could set my speaking back *fawty/fitty yeeuz.*

3

BEEP BEEP

My mother called me on a Wednesday night and told me to take the Friday afternoon train home. It would leave Lancaster, Pennsylvania, late enough so I wouldn't miss classes, but would arrive in New York early enough for dinner. *We need to talk.*

Almost five decades later, I still remember the tempered, level tone of her voice when she said that. There was no theatrical command that I *get home NOW*, no customary blend of accents. Even the concept that we would *talk* rather than that I would *shut up and listen* was strange. So I asked if she felt all right. She told me *Don't be stupid* and then, instead of good-bye, took a deep breath, added *Get a one-way ticket*, and hung up.

That one-way-ticket business was alarming. I was eighteen, a freshman at Franklin and Marshall College, finally not living at home, and there was no way I wasn't coming back to campus on Sunday night. And traveling by train. Because there was also no way I'd agree to a three-and-a-half-hour Sunday drive to Lancaster with my mother and her new boyfriend, Julius. If necessary, I was prepared to walk the 144 miles.

I met them, as agreed, outside Penn Station. Hunched in her mink coat, a Chesterfield pinched in her raised left hand, my mother frowned as she opened the passenger door and leaned forward so I could squeeze into the back seat of Julius's eleven-year-old Nash Rambler, which looked like an aardvark. The windows were closed against the winter air and the hot interior was dense with smoke. After quick hellos, no one spoke until we cleared the Queens Midtown Tunnel. Then, as he drove toward Long Island in lightly swirling snow, Julius started turning around to make polite, quick eye contact with me as he uttered each phrase: *There's something. I need. To ask you. Okay?*

This was even more uncharacteristic than my mother's subdued tone on the phone. The few times I'd been together with them, Julius had barely spoken. And when he had, my mother archly silenced him. Or made fun of his elocution and hesitant manner. *His name's not F-fwoyd, you silly man.* Now she was not only letting him talk, she wasn't criticizing him for failing to keep his eyes on the road.

I'd been sure my mother planned to demand, yet again, that I transfer to a college near home. And since I couldn't imagine her convincing this kindly man, whom she'd met only three months earlier, to serve as an intermediary, I was confused about what was going on, what he might be permitted to ask me. He couldn't be after my opinion about having Chinese food for dinner because my mother made all restaurant decisions without input. Maybe he wanted to know the quickest way to Long Beach, where my mother lived. But, grave and unsmiling, his thick glasses flashing light, the gentle sixty-three-year-old postal service manager then proceeded to ask me for her hand in marriage. *We want your blessing.*

§

The idea, so formal and correct, old-fashioned, respectful of me and my mother and of marriage, must have been Julius's. I noticed that he'd dressed in a suit and tie. It may have been the winter of *The Sounds of Silence* and "19th Nervous Breakdown," at the heart of the 1960s, but Julius was creating a Frank Sinatra, Tommy Dorsey Band, 1940s scene there in the Rambler.

All of which explained my mother's uncharacteristic behavior. She didn't ask anyone for permission or for blessing, including God. Her preferred approach would have been to announce her plans, tell me to call Julius and congratulate him, and instruct me to write a brief speech, to be delivered at their wedding, in praise of the treasure he was getting. So Julius must have insisted on including me at this stage. I can't imagine how he got her to agree, but it was obvious that she wasn't pleased by the scene, especially since she'd been reduced to an extra in it.

As she sat there staring at the road ahead, I restrained myself from shouting *YES! SHE'S YOURS!* and also from laughing with delight. This was what they'd summoned me home for? I could have blessed them by phone and stayed on campus to write the paper due early next week on Henry James's *Washington Square*. Which, come to think of it, was also a strange tragicomedy of manners about curious courtship, and what happened when a suitor's request for a woman's hand was denied by her father. I was hardly going to deny Julius's request, but the situation inside the car was clearly in earnest. No cackling. I needed to be taking this seriously.

The prospect of my mother's remarriage thrilled me. She'd been a widow since my father's sudden death in 1961. For nearly five years, we'd lived together in a tiny beachfront apartment, each struggling to find our ways separately and together. It was a volatile mix, and I'd been deeply relieved to escape to Lancaster, dreading each trip home from college, crammed together again with my mother's misery. Now, I thought, she would be Julius's to worry about.

In the brief pause, as he continued darting glances toward the back seat, Julius may have thought me hesitant to approve his proposal. That was when he offered me his car, as a kind of dowry.

Julius's grown children had called his car "the Cigar." The Rambler was a stubby, tubular, two-door, white sedan that made a lot of noise as it burrowed through traffic. The engine hacked and had an asthmatic undergrumble, the steering wheel squealed when it was turned, the arched brake pedal rebounded with a dramatic thump whenever it was released from duty. Above fifty miles an hour, the car began to tremble as though in fear of what might be asked of it next. The seat coverings were all cracked and, in the back, disgorging innards. It smelled like my mother's cigarettes. Julius was having trouble keeping the windshield clear inside or out. Maybe it wasn't the most elegant of dowries, but I was prepared to accept the deal.

Almost nineteen, I'd come of age to a rock 'n' roll soundtrack that featured Ronny & the Daytonas and their little GTO, with its *three deuces and a four-speed and a 389,* or the Beach Boys and their little deuce coupe, with its *four-speed dual quad posi-traction 409.* On the few occasions when I'd thought about the kind of car I might like to own, I'd certainly imagined myself in something sportier than this little ninety-horsepower Nash Rambler with its *Hydra-Matic 184* and optional heater.

As we drove through increasing snowfall, I couldn't stop hearing the tiny bicycle-horn toot from the 1958 novelty song "Beep Beep," a sound that had been intended to represent a *little Nash Rambler,* stuck in second gear, as it chased after a Cadillac. *The guy must have wanted to pass me out / As he kept on tooting his horn (beep beep).* That record by the Playmates, which made it to number four on the charts, had helped render Nash Ramblers forever silly, the toy poodle of the auto world, a mockery of everything that might be hip about a car. Even the cartoon roadrunner's beep was more manly. Since the age of eleven, the Playmates' version had been my image of the vehicle I was now about to inherit.

Still, I was elated by the idea of possessing any car of my own. And as I considered the problem of the car's image, I thought it was possible to adjust my angle of view, to see a '55 Rambler as a real improvement over the cars I'd driven before.

In high school driver's education class, I'd been taught in a 1958 Edsel Citation, with its huge horsecollar-shaped grille, taillights like gulls' wings, and push-button *teletouch* automatic-transmission controls, which were located at the center of the steering wheel hub where a horn should be. One of my classmates had shifted the car into Neutral while trying to honk. Massive, ambitious, full of irrelevant design details, cumbersome to drive, the Edsel was a mastodon that had become extinct after only three years. The Rambler was a kind of anti-Edsel, small in all the ways an Edsel was large. It was compact, sensible, built to share rather than dominate the road, and its face was almost demurely downturned instead of raised like a bully's. It scooched rather than swaggered down the road. The Rambler stressed economy and restraint, lacking the decorative chrome, fancy fins, wide wheelbase, high style, bulked-up engine, power, luxury, or flash that characterized late 1950s and 1960s automobile construction.

It was what it was, unlike the Edsel, which was a Ford dressed for a costume party. My Rambler—it was time to start thinking of it that way—was a safe song rather than aggressive rock 'n' roll, was Nat King Cole singing about Route 66, not Wilson Pickett doing "Mustang Sally" or Janis Joplin wanting a Mercedes-Benz. Besides, my Rambler was a good fit for me, since I was stubby myself, and my body would be in harmony with my car's body. I'd felt swallowed while driving the Edsel, and needed a pillow to see over its steering wheel.

It was also possible, though remotely, to see my Rambler as a step up from the battered, dying Volkswagen Karmann Ghia that my aunt once let me take on solo jaunts through the upstate New York countryside. She'd simply handed me the keys, drawn a sketch on a cocktail napkin to give me a general idea of how standard transmissions worked, and told me to be careful. Who cared that its doors wouldn't open from the inside or that it had a lingering odor of largemouth bass? The Ghia might have been sportier, but by the time I was behind its wheel it was a rattletrap whose racket made pedestrians stop and stare. Or maybe they stared because of the lurching, or the clunking and grinding noises the car made, as I learned how to operate a clutch and gear shift.

My Rambler was certainly better than the rusted, salt-cankered, farting, 1960 Plymouth Fury my mother had owned and occasionally allowed me to borrow when I was a desperate high school senior. That car combined the Edsel's vast size and outrageous design with the Ghia's decrepitude and my mother's restrictive rules to symbolize everything that irritated me about cars. Aptly named, the Fury also retained a miasma of leftover rage from my mother's time behind the wheel, where she would scream abuse at other drivers or at road signs that had the audacity to tell her what to do—Stop or Yield—or not to do—Park or Enter. I fully understood why Stephen King chose a Fury to be the title character of his 1983 automobile horror story, *Christine.*

It was also better than the first car I'd ever had a serious relationship with, a 1953 Packard Clipper hardtop, which ran me over in the fall of 1954, when we lived in Brooklyn. I was seven and had raced between parked cars onto Lenox Road, fleeing from one of my mother's beatings. What I remember most clearly is the sound of the Packard's horn, a blare rather than a Rambler's timid beep beep. Packards meant business, and this one's right front corner knocked me backward and sideways against the trunk of a parked Studebaker, under which I then rolled and planned to remain until such time as everything stopped trying to hurt me. The driver was an off-duty policeman who sat on his bumper and cried. He said I'd come outta nowhere. He said I showed up like a friggin fawn onna country road. Bruised, cut, concussed, I spent the next week in bed, and still have dreams of veering looming screeching braying big cars.

I wasn't the only member of my family to be damaged by cars. In 1958, two cars conspired to cripple my father. His Buick had a flat tire in heavy traffic on Rockaway Boulevard during the dawn commute. He pulled onto the right shoulder, failing to notice the turn-out available for such purposes thirty feet ahead. He shut off the lights, leaving the car in semidarkness less than a yard from the road's edge. Apparently he didn't know how to change a tire, because he then dodged across six lanes of traffic to a stranger's home, where he called the AAA for assistance. Instead of waiting in a safe place for help to arrive, he dodged traffic again, walked behind his car, turned his back to oncoming traffic, and began to open the trunk. He was hit by a car that hopped the curb and slammed into him, flinging his chest into the still unopened trunk, shattering both legs between the bumpers. Emergency room doctors thought he would surely die. But after nearly a year in hospitals and two surgeries, he came home to finish convalescing. He was able to use crutches and a wheelchair to get around, then a built-up shoe and cane. Never again in the two years before his death did he walk normally.

Cars had tried to kill my brother, too, even smallish ones like his white Plymouth Valiant, which plowed into the wall of a deli. According to my brother, the car had taken control once it sensed that he was tired. It rammed the back of a Chevy stopped at a traffic light, darted left and accelerated, then took out a fire hydrant on the corner as it headed toward the deli. Only a raised cellar door protruding a few feet from the wall slowed the impact and saved his life. A few years later, a runaway Pontiac Le Mans tried the same late-night stunt, this time tangling first with a dump truck, which stopped the Le Mans cold.

But now I was about to own a kind, well-behaved, approachable car of my own, and I was ready for it. Before we'd gotten to the restaurant and begun celebrating my mother's engagement to Julius, I'd convinced myself that the Rambler was an excellent vehicle for me. Couldn't wait to have its keys in my hand. I finally owned a car! One whose symbolic connection with my mother's remarriage marked a shift of responsibility away from the life I'd lived with her and toward the life I was beginning to shape for myself.

I also began to appreciate what a gift Julius had given me: not just a symbol, but the actual vehicle by which I could drive more fully out of my mother's life and into my own. It was as though I'd been given passage to a new world, a world in which there were no more demands that I move back home or transfer to a new college, no more pressure to spend summers sleeping on the fold-out couch in my mother's den. It had happened so fast, like an attentive God's answer to a fervent prayer, that I could only laugh. By morning, all the snow had melted.

ᔕ

Odd as it may seem, Nash Ramblers were a product of grand innovation and visionary thinking, a triumph of American zeal. At first, though, it seemed the antithesis of what our supercharged post–World War II consumers wanted.

Charles W. Nash created Nash Motors in 1916, after resigning as president of General Motors. In 1937, to survive the Depression, Nash merged with an appliance manufacturer, Kelvinator, famous for its refrigerators. Not surprisingly, the company soon introduced an optional air-conditioning and hot-water heating system in its cars. Inventive, competitive, they also introduced such features as the bed-in-a-car, reclining seats, mass-produced unibody construction, and *airflyte* design to improve gas mileage.

According to a 1958 *Time* magazine article, Nash-Kelvinator's then-president George Mason decided in 1950 that Americans were "ready to return to basic transportation and a smaller, compact car."

Despite the ongoing popularity of long, low, wide cars laden with chrome and fins and V-8 engines, Mason and his successor—the soon-to-be U.S. presidential candidate George Romney—were convinced that compact cars would claim a significant niche in the emerging automobile market. They introduced the first Rambler and "drove it into the field, where the only competition was foreign."

This prototypical compact, made for the steel-short, strapped American economy, was so successful that Romney was soon able to pay off his company's bank debts of nearly thirty-four million dollars. It was Romney who coined the phrase *gas-guzzling dinosaurs* to position the Rambler in an automobile market dominated by super-size designs. The timing was exquisite, anticipating the Interstate Highway Act of 1956, which made long-distance driving more feasible and gas economy more vital, and the impending growth of suburban life, which made owning a car more essential.

Early Ramblers wore long skirts: their front and back wheels were hidden within the car's exterior, enclosed for better dynamics, creating an unusually low-slung body with a squatty profile, tires peeking out modestly, like ankles. The design was unusual, especially for the way it enveloped the front wheels, and the impression that a sharp turn might bring wheel and body into contact. Rounded and humped, almost cylindrical at the snout, scooting along close to the ground, Ramblers really did resemble aardvarks. In long skirts.

In 1954, when Nash-Kelvinator merged with the Hudson Motor Car Company to form American Motors Corporation, Nash Ramblers were in their final days. My 1955 model was the first to hike its skirts and reveal the front wheels. It was also the last to utilize the old two-door, short-wheelbase design. Things were changing at Nash-Kelvinator, and with their compact car, and soon the Rambler would become an American Motors brand altogether. But within the narrow limits of a car that didn't pay much attention to style, the particular model I owned was about as stylish as a Nash Rambler ever got. Despite my doubts, I was driving a once-avant-garde vehicle.

§

I knew none of that history. I'd never had an interest in car design or mechanics, was never a car aficionado. As a boy, what excited me most about cars was noting the various colors of their steering wheels. *Look! A red one!* I also collected sightings of license plates from as many states as possible, once scoring a rare New Mexico on the streets of Brooklyn. But engines, design features, performance values? Not my world.

Perhaps my father's approach to cars, before his injuries, was responsible for my limited perspective: he simply bought a new black Buick, with black steering wheels, every two years, and seldom talked about them. Well, once he came home wildly excited over a new model's feature allowing him to set a speed-limit warning. It would buzz if he exceeded, say, thirty-five, and I still remember his laughter when he took us out for a blistering dash down Church Avenue in Brooklyn to demonstrate.

Lack of interest in cars was unusual for a boy growing up when I did, when cars were near the cultural and even psychological center of things for so many males. In her book *As Seen on TV: The Visual Culture of Everyday Life in the 1950s*, Karal Ann Marling devotes a substantial chapter to "Autoeroticism: America's Love Affair with the Car in the Television Age." She writes at length about the popular position of cars at that time, the way "the lunkers, the dreamboats, the befinned, bechromed, behemoths . . . lurked in the driveways of several million brand new ranch houses in the suburbs" and how, watching typical families on television, "in prime time, the nation aspired to the conditions of these golden, godlike creatures in their insolent chariots."

Not me. I aspired to the conditions of golden, godlike creatures on a baseball diamond or football field. I collected, played, and tinkered with sports cards, not cars, not trucks. At nineteen, I knew almost nothing about automobile mechanics or operation except how to drive. I could also get a car filled with gas, have its oil level checked, and replenish the air in its tires. What I'd learned in driver's ed about pistons and gears and chassis was quickly forgotten. I had a few fantasies, fired by those great rock songs, but no essential, soulful connection to cars. To me, cars were for transportation, and driving was a task to be completed safely, efficiently, as when I drove a dump truck one summer for the landscape contractor who employed me.

ॐ

Since freshmen were prohibited from having cars on campus, after driving my Rambler back to Lancaster I did what most of my class-mates did: stashed it on various side streets during the remaining three months of my first academic year. I trundled it out for the few dates I was lucky enough to have, rare events since the college was still three years away from becoming coeducational. One of my dates was with a rebellious young Mennonite woman from Lancaster County who hadn't quite shaken her phobia of cars, particularly of their chrome, which reflected a forbidden view of the human face. Fortunately, there was so little chrome on my car, and its white paint job was so dull, that she wasn't at risk. A blind date, imported from New York for a weekend, arrived by train and walked with me from the station to the car joking about the jalopy her brother had just bought, a goofy '55 Rambler that made her doubt his masculinity. Our weekend never recovered from her first glance at my car.

I had little success using cars as a setting for seduction. During a holiday break earlier that year, before getting the Rambler, I'd had a date with a former high school classmate who'd just been named a finalist for Miss George Washington University. We parked my mother's Fury in a small nook behind the Long Beach tennis courts and talked across the vast front seat for a while. Then we moved closer together, and after a few kisses she whispered that we couldn't go further because I would inevitably fall in love with her, only to be left heartbroken. I suppose I invited such treatment, being with her in my Mommy's car, which had to be home before ten. My Rambler didn't turn out to be any more conducive to romance. Little wonder that, for me, cars long remained nothing more than tools for transportation.

Unreliable, often dangerous tools, through my twenties. Of course, if I'd taken proper responsibility, and learned or relearned a few basic principles about car maintenance, things might have been different. Within six months, the Rambler's brakes began to fail. I had to push the pedal farther and farther toward the floorboard to slow the car down, but it didn't occur to me to have the problem checked. One evening in Long Beach, no matter how hard I stomped, there was no braking action at all. Applying gradual upward pressure to the hand-controlled emergency brake, running a few red lights with my horn tooting (*his horn went beep beep beep*), I drove the flat streets until the car slowed enough to stop against a parking meter without causing much damage.

I didn't believe that Julius had been planning to kill me by passing along a car he knew to be dangerous. He was horrified by what happened. But I still find myself considering the metaphoric implications of his gift to me. A hand-me-down car with an aging body and hidden faults in return for my mother's fifty-six-year-old hand in a second, soon-to-be-harrowing marriage. A scrappy little vehicle that, appreciated in a certain way, appreciated with a long view and a sociological overlay, suggested that small was beautiful. An old-fashioned car, a model soon to be discontinued, able to go but not able to stop. I also still think about the plot possibilities for a mystery novel in which the new husband gives his annoying stepson a gift that would soon threaten the young man's life. Maybe the stepson would die and the mother be stimulated to revenge. Nah. Or the stepson survive and seek revenge, upping the ante with an equally threatening gift. Also nah. I recognized Julius's gift for what it was: a kind, generous gesture of embrace from a man who was going to become my stepfather.

It was feasible to have the brakes repaired. But by the time they failed, there was enough wrong with my Rambler to make getting rid of it a more attractive option. Maybe someone who appreciated cars and the virtues of a Rambler would want to take it into the seventies. I placed an ad in the Lancaster newspaper and was contacted by a young woman, a nurse at St. Joseph's Hospital, whose father had owned four Nash automobiles and had taught her to drive on a '55 Rambler. Father and daughter arrived on campus together, inspected the car for a half hour, and agreed to my price on the spot.

Then, with a little financial help from Julius and my mother, I bought a stripped-down 1966 two-door Ford Falcon coupe. The cheapest option I could find for a brand-new car, it had a standard transmission with the gear-shift lever mounted on the shaft of the steering wheel, a radio, plastic seats, and an ample trunk. To this day, that Falcon is the loudest car I ever owned, with floorboards perhaps thinner than my fingernail. It was a soft pastel color my mother called baby blue, Julius called sky blue, and my Mennonite girlfriend called light cyan.

That was the car in which I moved to southern Illinois for graduate school, gaining still more distance from home. One day, three years after I bought the Falcon, I stopped for gas along the Pennsylvania Turnpike, returning from a visit to Baltimore. I asked the service station attendant to check my oil and water, then pulled back onto the turnpike, accelerating to sixty, and the hood—which had not been properly closed—flew open and wrapped itself around my windshield, blinding me just as the road turned. I managed to lean far enough out of the window to see my way over to the shoulder, where I stopped and leaned back in my seat until breath returned.

The hood had to be hammered back down toward flatness, though it retained all sorts of waves and wrinkles, then wired to its latch. Never properly closed, it would lift and howl threateningly in the headwind. I drove on to school, keeping the speed under forty for the next nine hundred miles across Pennsylvania, West Virginia, Ohio, Indiana, and Illinois.

Part Two

On and Off the Page

4

PLAYING THE COCK

Th' Cock's comin'! . . . Into your houses, shut to th'
windows, bar th' doors!

Sean O'Casey,
from *Cock-a-Doodle Dandy*

For two weeks in the winter of 1968 I spent my evenings as the incarnation of erotic power. I was *a lifesize dancing figure of fertility and
sexual temptation, the dark prophet of the life force, the proud prancing
Cock* who embodied *the sex-call, the active spirit, the sheer joy of living.*
I was a *badass bird* who *seduces the women, alienates the men, and
precipitates a crisis of community morals.*

It was exhausting work. I lost ten pounds. Covered in bruises and
rashes, I shed feathers, smelled funky, couldn't sit down because my
tail was too stiff and long. My face itched but I couldn't scratch it
because of how my wings worked. After the first week, my shanks
sagged and I stepped on my spurs when I whirled. I had a sore throat
but still had to *crow with sexual urgency.*

Here's what I was supposed to look like: *He is of a deep black plumage, fitted to his agile and slender body like a glove on a lady's hand; yellow feet and ankles, bright-green flaps like wings, and a stiff cloak falling like a tail behind him. A big crimson crest flowers over his head, and crimson flaps hang from his jaws. His face has the look of a cynical jester.* I did have the prescribed *huge, handsome crimson comb*, and was yellow from hock to claw, but my wings weren't green. They matched my black plumage and that plumage puffed far out from my body, more like an umpire's chest protector than a lady's glove. My yellow beak blinded me when I jumped or turned my head.

Ꭳ

To boost my spirits, the director who cast me said the Cock was the title role in the play. The lead. But the leading actor in Sean O'Casey's 1949 play, *Cock-a-Doodle Dandy*, is a big rooster, described by an O'Casey biographer, Garry O'Connor, as *the beautiful and effective symbol of the cock who says nothing, only crows: the Lord of Misrule, the pagan Oisin*. He is an *expressionistic device*, the epitome of *those instinctive and creative urges which men suppress at their peril*. O'Casey himself said the Cock symbolizes *the desire of man for a woman and the desire of woman for the desire of man*.

I had no lines to speak, only—according to the stage directions— a mixture of sometimes *lusty*, sometimes *short and sharp*, or *violent and triumphant*, or *loud exultant*, or *mighty* crows. Also some *cackling with a note of satisfaction, even victory in it*. I had to master the nuanced cock-crow and cackle.

I also had to dance and prance, perform a goose-step march, glide and weave around various obstacles and people, spring over walls, run atop narrow, steeply sloped stone fences, pirouette, appear out of nowhere and vanish back into it. I had to sprint directly toward the audience and stop in a flash without skidding off the stage. I had to transform into a tall hat. Wearing a bulky forty-pound costume with a heavy tail and slippery cock-footed yellow tights, with my hands strapped to flapping-sticks sewn inside long wings, and with that blinding beak, I had to portray the glory of erotic power. Had to be *a human sized bird-like creature exuding grace and sexual energy.*

ⓢ

This was not how I saw my career as an actor progressing. I was a junior at Franklin and Marshall College, and *Cock-a-Doodle Dandy* was my second role in the school's acclaimed Green Room Theatre, which has spawned such stage and film professionals as James Lapine, Roy Scheider, Franklin J. Schaffner, and Treat Williams. In the fall, I'd played Pompey in Shakespeare's *Measure for Measure* and fancied myself, with no basis in reality, as a promising young comic actor possessing an as-yet untapped capacity to play romantic or dramatic heroes. Being cast as the Cock did little to encourage such fancies. Though it was a role that would be performed the next year on Broadway by Barry Bostwick, who went on to originate the role of Danny Zuko in *Grease* and win a Tony award, and though it would also be played at Dublin's Abbey Theatre by a woman, the Irish television star Martina Stanley, I failed to see its transformative possibilities. Upon learning that I was to play the Cock, I felt humiliated and thought about quitting. After all, I had a full load of classes to deal with and a daily job as the reader for the chairman of the English Department, who was blind. Did I really need to add six weeks of nightly rehearsals to my schedule? To play a speechless, screeching Cock?

With the cast—jittery and unsure of this strange, farcical play— scattered in seats throughout the theater, I opened the first read-through with a cackle that, apparently, sounded more like a chicken's chattery squawk than a cock's lusty crow. Everyone laughed, and I remember thinking *that's it, I'm done.* But in the next moments, I realized that the mood had shifted, the cast seemed more relaxed and high spirited. I'd gotten the sound wrong, but I could already see that the Cock's weird presence might have power over the proceedings. Still, did it have to be me?

Afterward, the director sat next to me in the theater's front row and put his arm around my shoulder. He looked at the empty stage rather than at me, as if to focus my imagination on the work ahead, and told me playing the Cock would be excellent for my development as an actor. *Be a Brilliant Bird!* Also, since I'd been a ballplayer, I could think of this as playing out of position for the good of the team. *Put on the mask!* He said I needed to go out and do some field work so I could come up with a better cock-crow, but shouldn't even consider quitting. And then he said the sort of thing I would hear, in various manifestations, for the next two months: *rise to the challenge, oh Cock.*

As part of my next-great-star fantasy, I'd been reading about Method Acting. How would Marlon Brando approach the role of the Cock? I needed to immerse myself in cockness! That would, according to the theory, let me find the emotions and memories required to manifest pure sexual joy in every movement and sound. Unfortunately, at age twenty I was in need of further research in this area. When the director had ordered me to conduct fieldwork, I knew he didn't mean what I wanted him to mean. He meant I should get up before dawn, drive out to the Amish farmland around Lancaster, where the theater was located, and listen to cocks greet the morning. It seems that remembering the sound of cooped chickens in my father's kosher poultry market would not be adequate preparation.

ᘓ

Cock-a-Doodle Dandy is a play about the consequences of sexual repression. A critic reviewing a recent production in Scotland called it "one great rumbustious raspberry in the face of the whole creeping pack of whingeing, hypocritical busybodies, terminal, superstitious stick-in-the-muds and thin-lipped moral guardians." O'Casey himself said it was "a secular hymn to life."

The play is set in the small village of Nyadnanave, which means "nest of saints" but sounds like it means "nest of knaves," a place where being joyful or exuberant, especially in matters of desire, is considered sinful, threatening, evil. Where men believe "a woman's always a menace to a man's soul. Woman is th' passionate path to hell!" The plot is simple: The Cock materializes at various places in the village, his actions spreading disorder and disruption, leading to outbreaks of wild dancing and flirtation and kissing and drink-fueled licentiousness. Altar lights and holy pictures are damaged. Removing him becomes the local priest's obsession. Driven out at last, the Cock departs along with all the village women, one of whom declares as she leaves: "a whisper of love in this place bites away some of th' soul!"

Most of the male characters are terrified of the Cock. They hide from him, cast spells, consider him a demon, utter elaborate nonsensical curses against him (*ubique ululanti cockalorum ochone, ululo!*), try to kill or capture or drive him out of town. Tormented by his sudden appearances on their property or inside their homes, they fear "th' cock rampant in th' disthrict, desthroyin' desire for prayer, desire for work, an' weakenin' th' authority of th' pastors and masters of your souls!" Their talk only serves to ratchet up one another's anxiety: "Big powers of evil, with their little powers, an' them with their littler ones, an' them with their littlest ones, are everywhere."

The female characters, along with one male character—a singing, dancing charmer known as the Messenger—embrace the Cock's presence. "There's no harm in him beyond gaiety an' fine feelin'." They invite him to appear, offer to hang a wreath of roses around his neck, seek to protect him from harm, dance with him. They also realize that the Cock is a bringer of light into the gloom of their lives: "th' place'll lose its brightness if th' Cock's killed." The women are all horny and eager ("only to see his face again, only to hear him crow!" one chants). The great Cock unleashed in their midst completes them in a way nothing else in their lives seems to.

So it was up to me to trigger and affirm desire by personifying carnal energy. While dressed in a chicken suit. This was not a comic role, though the play was a comedy and it was easy to laugh at a giant rooster and his capers.

It was also up to me to oppose the chief source of repression in the play: the Catholic Church in Ireland. Me, the Kosher Cock, against Father Domineer, the church's representative in the village, and also against the terrified male residents called "oul' life-frighteners" by one of the feisty female characters. My function was to counter the darkness and heaviness of repression. My cavorting and cawing, and the way people reacted to it, revealed *a malignant sickness at the heart of modern society* and *exposed a theocratic community driven to hysteria by puritanical leadership*. I couldn't very well do that timidly.

After that pep talk from the director, I went to the library and read up on cocks' crowing, then drove into the countryside to hear them in person. What I discovered from my reading was that no one really knows why cocks crow. It may be a territorial declaration, or a warning to intruders seeking to damage the flock, or a cry of authority. It may be a response to rising light, even though a cock's crowing isn't confined to dawn. What I discovered from listening to the actual sound was that it tends to be four rather than five syllables (er-er er ER, rather than COCK-a-doodle do), and seems to come from the bird's whole body, not just the throat.

As I drifted past farms and heard the cocks, I thought about how to use what I'd learned. What was my territory in the play? Sure, the town of Nyadnanave, its life-force choked, its inhabitants thwarted. Also, and more particularly, the women living there—my flock—whom I both claimed and needed to protect. But it was more than that, too. I was claiming and protecting the joy of natural expression, with the cock-crow and cocky dance representing passion, appetite, creative energy. I was there to provoke, to show up wherever I wished—fields, yards, kitchens, bedrooms. If I crowed in response to rising light, it was the rising that mattered. The Cock was all about rising. After listening to the cacophony of cock-crows, I thought of the sound as song: these were birds, after all, and their raucous chorus was nothing less than an anthem of joy over another day in which to be strutting and bringing cockness to life. Better work on those loud, lusty, exultant crowings.

ṣ

We were staging the play at a time—early 1968—when the spirit of the Cock seemed rampant everywhere. The Beatles were singing *Why don't we do it in the road!* This was the time of *Hair: The American Tribal Love-Rock Musical* and John Updike's *Couples*, of the sex-crazed cartoon character Fritz the Cat, and the seductive Mrs. Robinson. As Morris Dickstein says in *Gates of Eden: American Culture in the Sixties*, "There's no question that the period saw dramatic changes in American sexual behavior—above all in public sexual expression—and especially in the younger generation."

Our rehearsals for *Cock-a-Doodle Dandy* began only four months after the Summer of Love ended, when over a hundred thousand young people gathered in San Francisco's Haight-Ashbury neighborhood to celebrate sex, drugs, and rock 'n' roll. In *1968: The Year That Rocked the World*, Mark Kurlansky writes of the larger culture's widespread impression "that these young people were having a lot of sex. Sex was now called 'free love,' because, with the pill, sex seemed free of consequences." In *Hippies: A Guide to an American Subculture*, Micah L. Issitt says, "Within the culture, sexuality was cast in a new light as the hippies rebelled against the 'dirty' or 'shameful' view of sex while promoting sex as the ultimate expression of unity, compassion, and love . . . something to be celebrated rather than hidden." Singer-songwriter-poet-novelist Leonard Cohen remembers the sixties this way: "If any two people had any kind of sexual affinity for each other they had to sleep with each other immediately, otherwise it was a terrible betrayal and waste."

According to Annie Gottlieb in her book *Do You Believe in Magic?*, "the Love Generation" believed "we could recapture the animal innocence of the body." She says, "In the compressed lexicon of the Sixties, love-making was like hitch-hiking, one of those all-purpose gestures." If it's true, as Philip Larkin declares in his poem "Annus Mirabilis," that "Sexual intercourse began / In nineteen sixty-three," then it came of age in 1968.

But not with noticeable effect at Franklin and Marshall College. Mine would turn out to be the last all-male class in the college's two-hundred-year history, with the first women admitted the year after we graduated. We were also among the first classes for which morning chapel attendance was no longer mandatory. Franklin and Marshall was a tradition-bound place, huddled on two hundred acres in conservative Lancaster, and it encountered sixties licentiousness gingerly. Our well-behaved, sparsely attended "be-in," cited in a recent history of the college as a prime example of a campus counterculture's emergence in the sixties, took place in Buchanan Park on the campus's south end, a small patch named after the only bachelor U.S. president. There were a few arrests for drug possession. I remember seeing a few couples holding hands under the glowering statue of Buchanan. One classmate lay on a blanket beside his young bride, sharing a slice of shoofly pie. We had the drugs and rock 'n roll, but not so much the sex.

Which is why I initially became involved in the Green Room Theatre. I hadn't been having anywhere near the amount of sex that the era of free love promised, or that I desperately wanted. If you weren't in a fraternity, if you didn't have a girlfriend back home somewhere, the theater was one of the few places to meet women because, when a play required actresses, the directors had to recruit them from the Lancaster community. I was, two years after arriving on campus, finally starting to date: a woman in the cast.

So things were lining up. If I looked at it properly, as a surprise, a challenge, an opportunity, playing the Cock may have been exactly the role I needed.

§

There's a Wikipedia page dedicated to *Cock-a-Doodle Dandy*. It describes the play as "a darkly comic fantasy in which a magic cockerel appears in the parish of Nyadnanave." But a cockerel is a young rooster, and the Cock in O'Casey's play doesn't seem young, a kid jazzed up on hormones and high spirits. He's savvier than that, experienced enough to vary his tactics, sophisticated enough for O'Casey to see him as *a cynical jester*. The Cock manages his great sexual energy for heightened effect rather than letting it run rampant. He's purposeful, a man in his prime rather than a rowdy adolescent, and that's how I would think of him. *Don't call me a cockerel!*

In rehearsal, I worked on maintaining various movements at the edge of control. I wanted my leaps and spins and loops to be as wild as I could make them without losing balance or missing a beat. There could be no flailing, wings waving in the air, no stumbling, no bumping into things. The Cock's antics had to be graceful. O'Casey's stage directions called for gliding and weaving, not stomping and storming. A dancer, not a fullback.

For weeks, I choreographed and practiced routines on the flat, empty stage until the set could be built. It would have sloped walls and fences with slender surfaces I needed to prance upon or leap over, a table and stools to avoid, and the rickety two-story facade of a house from whose windows and doors I needed to appear. Once the set was ready, any entrances, exits, and dance routines that weren't to be done on the stage's flat foreground had to be rechoreographed halfway through rehearsals to accommodate the narrow, angled spaces I'd now perform them on.

I worried about the way my moves had to keep being changed. I needed to practice what I was going to do, get the steps down, prepare myself so that it would all feel innate, because in performance the stage would be crowded with people and props, I was going to take up a lot of space, especially with my wings expanded, and I might not be able to see clearly.

Then, the day before dress rehearsal and three days before opening night, my costume arrived. Its sheer bulk plumped me up to 190 instead of 150 pounds, a 27 percent increase in the load my legs would carry. And my weight was now radically redistributed, altering balance. To achieve a rooster-like upper body, I wore a heavy, protruding rubbery coat, and my legs were encased in yellow tights and densely feathered knickers. A tail, stiff and thick and feathered, bent at ninety degrees and hanging all the way to the calves, protruded from my coccyx. I was like a gymnast whose work on the beam suddenly included a loaded backpack, shoulder pads, baby sling, and dangling whoopee cushion. The soles of my feet, covered in slick material, couldn't be relied on for traction. Seeing clearly might be the least of my problems.

The first time I ran down atop the sloped fence in costume, momentum carried me past the planned leap-off point. I landed in a heap on the stage with my tail sticking up and one wing trapped under my gut. I was unable to right myself. The director ran down the theater's aisle toward the stage yelling, "Somebody straighten up my cock."

The first time I attempted the goose-step late in scene 1, a march-like dance done in a trio with the concertina-playing Messenger and his beloved Marion in her naughty maid's costume, I raised my right leg as required and toppled over backward, taking Marion down with me. In scene 2, when I had to race onstage in complete darkness while a top hat got transformed into the Cock between flashes of lightning, I couldn't stop before smacking into a cluster of characters poised beside the house's front porch. In scene 3, "weaving a way between Mahan at the table, and Lorna, circling the garden," my feet went out from under me and I slid into the small round table like a runner stealing second base, sending it flying into the wings, stage left.

I was a danger to myself, the cast, the set. And, suddenly, a burden: because my hands were strapped to a stick inside the wings, enabling me to approximate a flapping motion and to hold the wings out stiffly, I could no longer climb the ladder backstage to access the house's upper story window from which I needed to thrust my head and issue "a violent and triumphant crow" in the middle of scene 1. A cast member, who was six foot eight and played the village's Sergeant, was recruited to lift me onto my perch.

I had two days in which to rechoreograph all twelve of my appearances onstage, incorporate them into everyone else's actions, and remember them well enough to help us all remain safe, in sync, and in character. I considered wearing my Cock's-head to class and on campus so I'd get accustomed to the limits of vision, but decided against it.

Then, a few days after the play opened, I came down with tonsillitis. This made crowing a serious challenge. Dancing too, in the heat of fever and stage lights and a forty-pound costume. When not needed onstage, I would take my Cock's-head off and wonder about the possibility of a Cock contracting tonsillitis. I didn't know at the time, but according to a website called "Poultry Community," chickens do actually have tonsils: "The pyloric tonsil is a novel peripheral lymphoepithelial organ of the gastrointestinal tract in the chicken. It forms a complete lymphoid ring at the beginning of the duodenum." This might have been a small comfort to me.

There was no understudy. For three days during the play's run, I was confined to the college infirmary, missing classes but allowed out for evening performances. The director visited every day at noon, and the Sergeant escorted me to the theater every evening at seven. And there, for ninety minutes a night, I went about my business as the incarnation of erotic power, that *badass bird, the dark prophet of the life-force.*

※

I loved playing the Cock. There was some lingering embarrassment when I moved among fellow students outside the theater, the concern that they thought my being cast as a rooster meant I wasn't a good enough actor to play a human. But I felt I'd overcome a range of physical and technical problems, found within myself a reservoir of resilience, and made a valuable contribution to the production by being irrepressible.

An old friend from the Green Room Theatre, the late Gary Blackton, once told me by e-mail that while he didn't remember much about our performances together in *Measure for Measure*, he did recall being in the audience for *Cock-a-Doodle Dandy.* "What I do remember is you as a rooster. Man, you had so much energy. That's what the play was about, the Irish Church's defeat of life-energy. And there you were, crouched in a corner, then jumping all around the stage, running on the walls, flapping your wings. You became the rooster, all right."

My roommate and best friend through those Green Room Theatre days, Lou Hampton, was one of the group's star performers. But he didn't take part in *Cock-a-Doodle Dandy*, and when I asked him this week what he recalled about my performance all those years ago, he said, "the only detail I remember from the play is you, standing on a wall."

What Gary and Lou recall may not sound like much, but in fact just being able to stand on that wall in my Cock regalia, and being able to communicate zest for life, turned out to be noteworthy accomplishments for me. I'd prepared to perform in one body but was required to perform, overnight, in another one instead. I'd found a spirit and emotional flexibility I didn't know I had.

Playing the Cock required me to put my body first, in typical sixties fashion. Make Body the foreground of my being, and liberate it from Mind. I needed to be nothing other than what I was in the moment onstage: a 190-pound Cock. This was astoundingly liberating for me, always so conscious and worried about my stubby body. And I was required to work with the body I had, the one I brought onstage, which was not the body my body and mind remembered from rehearsal, or even from the remaining hours of the day.

At the same time, playing the Cock taught me I couldn't always rely on my body, couldn't depend on it to remain as I knew it, from moment to moment, or to assume it would do what I wanted, or what it had done before. This turned out to be excellent preparation for what illness and aging demands of us across time.

Interviewed by the college newspaper shortly before opening night, the director said cast members "find opportunities in this particular play to make self-discoveries as actors and as individuals." This was the last thing I expected to be true of me as rehearsals began, and I found myself cast as a rooster. But *Cock-a-Doodle Dandy* was not, it turned out, so much about sexual liberation as it was about liberating the body itself.

I discovered, during those winter days in 1968, a different kind of life-force than I thought I was looking for in playing the Cock.

Though I found the one I was looking for too, with the woman I'd begun dating as rehearsals began. But I also found a core place in myself that I've come to associate with adaptability, the capacity to deal with sudden and unplanned-for obstacles, the sorts of challenges for which there is no relevant rehearsal. That's ultimately what made the Cock such a force, made him the epitome of those instinctive and creative urges that men suppress at their peril: his unquenchable passion to live fully, to do what he was called to do—his cocky, passionate dance—even as counterforces sought to still him.

5

THE BOTTOM SHELF

On Novels I Keep Trying and

Failing to Read

I love William Styron's novel *Sophie's Choice*. I've just never been able to finish reading it. Once, I got to page 312, a little more than halfway through the Vintage paperback edition. But usually I stop much sooner, unable to face yet another protracted scene of the paranoid schizophrenic Nathan Landau's crazed behaviors, vicious diatribes, escalating threats, devastating exits. I know these "mysterious vicissitudes of his mind and mood" are meant to be harrowingly dramatic, accumulating intensity and alarm as they foreshadow doom. They're meant to make readers feel what Nathan's targets feel, to make us identify with Nathan's abused, self-loathing Polish lover, Sophie Zawistowska, and the novel's overwhelmed narrator, Stingo. But for me the scenes just lose edge and interest as they recur two-three-four-five times, adding little about the characters, whose responses remain essentially unchanged. I get the point already.

Not only Nathan's eruptions but everything vital in the novel is pitched to extremes, a tonal and dramatic feverishness that soon becomes wearisome. Sophie's past and present degradations, for example, are relentlessly extravagant. Presented in fragmentary flashbacks, the wartime loss of her parents, husband, and way of life in Cracow; her arrest and deportation by the Nazis; her terrible experiences at Auschwitz are all relived in prolonged, close detail. I understand the intent, Styron's decision to provide maximum clarity about such awful events, and to personalize the Holocaust from the unfamiliar angle of a non-Jewish victim. But the flashbacks are slowly woven among scenes from the novel's present setting in which Sophie endures a hideous, public, faint-inducing humiliation in the Brooklyn College library followed by a grotesque New York subway molestation followed by utterly incapacitating illness and chiropractic mishandling along with Nathan's ongoing torments, Stingo's soaring lust, and adoration from her English teacher. The "beautiful body" she lugs around like a burden, and which so many male characters make demands upon, possesses a "sickish plasticity" and "sallowness," signs that it was "not wholly rescued from a terrible crisis." Early on, Stingo intrudes upon her privacy and sees her toothless face, further shattering Sophie's facade of balance. Meanwhile, as Styron doles out the misery, Stingo is repeatedly brought to shame in his most sensitive areas—his writing, sexual cravings, southern heritage, conflicting needs for fellowship and solitude—and even Stingo's father must get beaten up during a visit to New York.

Styron's compounding of fulsome calamity strains credibility, supersaturates my tolerance, numbs my responses, and, perhaps most problematic, diminishes what Sophie had endured under the Nazis by making it just one more among all the awful things, a matter of scale.

While my resistance to these scenes and dynamics escalates, so does the urge to skip yet another digressive backgrounder on the Nazis or on the history of the Old South. Stingo's familiar erotic fantasies and scarcely credible sexual encounters grow unendurable to read. Sophie's English farcically re-refalters, despite Styron's declaration that after her "first few months" in America "her difficulty with the language" was "soon overcome." Stingo stews and struggles and stews and struggles with his writing, fellow boarders step from the wings for needless cameos illustrating "the intense Jewishness of the little scene," narrative repetitions require Stingo to keep noting, "As I have said . . ." And I can't go on.

🌀

I recognize that my reaction to *Sophie's Choice* may be a bit off-kilter. After all, the novel is an enduring classic, ranked #96 in the Modern Library Board's list of 100 best novels of the twentieth century, and #57 on the Radcliffe Publishing Course's rival list. Amazon.com currently shows an average rating of four and a half out of a possible five stars posted by 186 readers.

But the experience of reading is at its best a passionate and quirky one, informed by all sorts of needs, expectations, experiences, prejudices, situations. I know that the way *Sophie's Choice* gets to me, then loses me, says at least as much about me as about the novel. I'm defeated by its excesses, though most readers are not, and though I realize that a preference for concision and understatement are essential qualities of my taste in fiction, I return to *Sophie's Choice* again and again. That's what gets me: I keep coming back. Because there's so much about the novel that appeals to me, especially when I'm not reading it, I delude myself into thinking I'll handle its flaws. This is irrational reading behavior, but I feel certain I'm not alone in it. There are strong personal forces at work when we choose what to read.

Sophie's Choice begins in the exact time, place, and milieu where I was born: summer of 1947 in Brooklyn's Flatbush neighborhood, which Stingo several times calls "the Kingdom of the Jews." I remember a house next to my Grandma Kate's that was just like Yetta Zimmerman's, where the novel's main characters live. It was painted a vivid yellow (instead of Yetta's pink), and filled with Morris Finks and Moishe Muskatblits and Lillian Grossmans, with Nathans and Sophies whose outbursts were easily audible and who would rush out the front door and dance down the stoop as they struggled into coats and spat angry parting remarks. I remember "the Church Avenue station of the BMT" right near that yellow house, and the neighborhood's "pickle-fragrant air."

The personal resonance of this setting attracts me deeply, and I always begin the novel with a joyful eagerness to experience Styron's sense of this familiar place. Especially as it was at the time I was born, which of course I can't remember. It's nearly a home movie. I yield to the opening passages with something like my full soul. "One of the pleasant features of that summer which I so vividly remember was the weather, which was sunny and mild, flower-fragrant, almost as if the days had been arrested in a seemingly perpetual springtime."

It's not that I need to identify so closely with a fictional world in order to engage with a novel, but rather that such a rare confluence of time and place adds a provocative layer to my interest as a reader, and further enriches the way fiction can illuminate a reader's life. So my entanglement with this novel has a serious private dimension, a characteristic that defines nearly all the novels I end up unable to stand but unable to resist, over and over.

Sophie's Choice is narrated with a mixture of nostalgia and horror by a mature writer looking back on his early twenties, when he was setting out on his first real writing project—a novel that would establish his name—and leaving behind the vividly sketched, heartless publishing industry where he'd been working. I'm enticed by this element as well, the writer and his shadowy experience across the years, the older writer making fictional use of his early writerly experience. As I age—I'm now sixty-six—the attraction intensifies.

Another lure is Stingo's powerful and positive connection with his father. I never had this with my own father, a man who was seldom home, who seldom spoke other than to command or to argue with his wife. Injured and dying so young, he was barely a presence in my life, and—especially once I reached Stingo's age and began to write—that presence was confined to a few memories. I can't recall the sound of his voice.

In *Sophie's Choice*, the letters sent to Stingo by his father, their affectionate and concerned tone, their kindness and engagement with Stingo's life, stir me. So do the old man's generous gifts, his consideration, the way his son's interests are paramount in his thoughts. I like, at least initially, the way they talk when Stingo's father comes to New York for a visit. The way they look out for each other. As with so much else in this novel, the father-son relationship grabs me and touches an emotional need that is at the heart of my enthrallment with fiction. But then it too begins to lose its draw as Styron drags things out, repeats, elaborates, lavishes more language on by-now-familiar material.

Perhaps because I'm so drawn to the novel, and love the way its world opens for me, I end up feeling betrayed. The narrative and characters, at first so compelling, are sabotaged by the narration and characterization. The story stagnates as Styron's authorial mannerisms, his elaborative style ("I began to do, or undergo, or experience what I believe is known as a slow burn") and riverine storytelling, become a barrier rather than a portal, and the novel's voice, so seductive and compelling, grates as it drones on. The aspects I most admire become the very things that put me off. I skim to see how the plot works out, then declare myself done.

What usually happens next is that I trade in my copy at a used bookshop, or recycle it if I've scribbled on the margins (*False! Overdone!*). Then a few years later, filled with enthusiasm, convinced that *this* time I will finish the novel, that I've moved beyond whatever made me lose patience last time and am ready again for Stingo's intimate presence, the Brooklyn setting that means so much to me, the intensity of emotion and character, I purchase a replacement copy and start all over. This is a process that has been going on for thirty years, since the novel first appeared and I bought it for $12.95 in its spare, off-white hardback edition with the brown writing on the cover. I believe I've tried to read *Sophie's Choice* five times now, and spent over a hundred dollars—adjusted for three decades of inflation—on a book I'm deeply drawn to but can't actually stand.

🌀

If I behaved like this only with *Sophie's Choice*, then I wouldn't have needed to devote an entire shelf to novels I keep trying and failing to read, keep disposing of, and keep repurchasing. Finally recognizing the pattern, I dedicated the bottom shelf of a small bookcase in my writing room to these books. So now I retain them after quitting on them, making it both easier and cheaper when, hopeful and determined, I need to start one again.

A couple of years ago, I bought a new copy of Boris Pasternak's *Doctor Zhivago*. Beverly and I had watched a rebroadcast of the 2002 Masterpiece Theatre production, starring Keira Knightley as Lara, had reminisced about the 1965 Julie Christie version, and, fired up by the love story, I thought *I'm ready to try that novel again.*

Highlighting my way through its opening chapter, I was moved by young Yuri Zhivago sobbing at his mother's fresh grave in the lashing cold and rain, then by his spooky first night in Uncle Nikolai's care. How could I have disliked such a vividly told story? But by the time I reached page 50, "the time of the Presnia uprising," I was done. Not a very thorough attempt, but enough to bring back all the reasons why I can't read this novel: a rickety, time-shifting structure; sketchy characterizations that border on caricature and include incredible personal transformations; sentimentality and mushy romance conventions; ridiculous coincidences; clunky symbolism; dull polemics. The author was far more present than his characters, his touch heavy, his style self-consciously poetic.

My first encounter with *Doctor Zhivago* took place in the winter of 1959, a few months after it appeared in English translation. Despite beginning with serious intention, I could only make it through about half the first chapter, stopping where Yuri's Uncle Nikolai has "gone through Tolstoyism and revolutionary idealism" as he "passionately sought an idea, inspired, graspable, which in its movement would clearly point the way toward change, an idea like a slash of lightning or roll of thunder capable of speaking even to a child, or an illiterate." This stuff was a little hard for me, and way too boring. I was eleven at the time.

I'd decided to read *Doctor Zhivago* in 1959 to save my father's life. A few months earlier, when he'd been critically injured in the car accident, I'd been told repeatedly that he might not survive, then that he might not walk. I wasn't permitted to visit him because hospital policy in those days assumed that a germ-riddled child might contaminate the entire ward, and my family wanted to spare me sight of his suffering. Unable to help, terrified by all I'd heard and imagined, I seized upon an opportunity when someone sent him a copy of *Doctor Zhivago* as a get-well gift.

I knew my father would never read it—all I'd ever seen him read was the evening newspaper as he sat in his easy chair and consumed butterscotch candies—so I decided reading *Doctor Zhivago* for him would be my job. After all, it was about a physician, a healer. Maybe I'd pick up some important medical information. On the flyleaf the gift-giver had drawn a cartoon of my father, glasses and characteristic cigar in place, standing with his trousers sagging around his ankles, his buttocks being examined by a doctor with a stethoscope who says, "You'll be good as new in no time, Mr. Skloot." It was as though the novel carried some sort of magical powers I might release by reading it, thereby making my father good as new.

But I couldn't, no matter how often I picked the book up and stared at its cover, that white dust jacket with purple and sky-blue squiggles meant to represent clouds looming above a snowy Russian landscape. There was a sleigh approaching a small house where bare trees and a rickety snow fence stand guard. The image was cold, threatening, a depiction of dangerous forces that don't care who you are, and of home as someplace very fragile. I put it safely on a shelf beside my World Book Encyclopedias.

I tried reading *Doctor Zhivago* again in the summer of 1965, during a three-month limbo between high school graduation and freshman year at college when I was eighteen and confined to bed with a reactivation of mononucleosis. My father had been dead for almost four years. While I knew my failure to read *Doctor Zhivago* hadn't really led to his death, I was always aware of the novel's presence, of a duty I felt toward it and my father, an enduring connection between them. I'd often taken the book down and set it beside my bed, knowing it was absurd to think this brought my father closer, not really intending to read it. But when I was sick, with little to do other than read, having completed the books assigned for freshman orientation and the gift books from my aunt (*The Man with the Golden Gun*, *Hotel*, *Up the Down Staircase*), no longer interested in the Hardy Boys, having few other books available in my mother's apartment, I thought of trying *Doctor Zhivago*.

What I remember most from that attempt was feeling horror that so many characters experienced sudden losses of, vanishings by, and partings from loved ones. Yuri's mother dies, his father commits suicide, he's yanked from his familiar life to travel with his uncle, and soon placed with yet another family, the Gromekos, all in the first two chapters. The heroine, Lara Guishar, has lost her father, and Yuri's new friend Misha Gordon is abandoned by his family. Even the country is coming apart, turning against itself as its various factions generate mayhem. Echoing all this mayhem is the way Pasternak introduces then discards so many characters and situations.

Though I identified with loss, and experienced the first parts of the novel in an intensely personal way, I think what thwarted me was a feeling of being manipulated. Sure, the story had some compelling elements, but it was also cluttered and felt overwrought, the emotions bogus. I hated the feeling that I couldn't trust the author, that in vast Russia you would routinely bump into people you knew, just like in my apartment building, and even people he told us were dead would come back later, utterly remade. My still-unformed aesthetic sensibility rebelled at the way this writer behaved, at the obstacles he placed in the way of credibility.

I think this was the period when my reading taste began to coalesce, and I clearly didn't like stories that struck me as feverish or melodramatic. I wanted emotional authenticity, no doubt prompted by witnessing my mother's hysteria close-up. And, especially in the case of certain books like *Doctor Zhivago*, which bore an almost talismanic significance for me, I took things personally.

Later that summer, a family friend named Sylvia, who also happened to be my doctor's wife, brought over a copy of Thomas Mann's *The Magic Mountain*. She told me it was about being sick and being cut off from your normal life because of it. Bam! Another special, talismanic book. The novel was thick as a brick, as was its prose, but I tried hard to get into the story because I didn't want to disappoint Sylvia or my doctor. I thought it moved as stiffly as Frankenstein, each sentence lurching along, the speeches awkward, the characters scarcely human. It looked and felt like a novel, it was made up of a novel's components, but I thought it was a fake, and it kept putting me to sleep. Maybe that was Sylvia's intent, via her husband, who kept saying that the best treatment for me was rest.

Four years later, having recovered from yet another recurrence of mononucleosis, having graduated from college as an English major and working toward a master's degree in English, I felt that my reading still had huge gaps, especially in foreign language literature. Between my first and second terms in grad school, I decided to start filling in those gaps, and found Sylvia's gift still on my shelves.

By this time in my life, I knew I wanted to be a writer, and had chosen Southern Illinois University in order to study with the Irish poet Thomas Kinsella. One evening at his house in Carterville, he asked what I was reading during the upcoming term break. When I said *The Magic Mountain*, his expression softened—a rare occurrence—and he said he envied me my first exposure to it, adding that he'd taught himself German as a young man in order to read the novel in its original language. Holy smoke! I decided not to tell him I'd tried and failed to read it before. In English.

Nor did I tell him later that I couldn't make it past the third day of Hans Castorp's seven-year stay at the International Sanatorium Berghof. If he asked how I was doing with the novel, I was prepared to say that I had so much other work to prepare for the next term's teaching and study, and was also working on a long poem, so I'd put *The Magic Mountain* aside. All of which was technically true, though I'd have kept reading it anyway if I hadn't hated being in the presence of Thomas Mann's voice.

Distant, formal, haughty, soulless, the narration pushed me away rather than lured me in. Mann seemed to condescend toward his characters, particularly the protagonist, the twenty-three-year-old engineer Hans Castorp, who comes across as a dull, limited presence. In a description that illustrates in style and attitude what bothered me most about his novel, Mann writes, "Castorp was neither a genius nor an idiot, and if we refrain from applying the word 'mediocre' to him, we do so for reasons that have absolutely nothing to do with his intelligence and little or nothing to do with his prosaic personality, but rather out of deference to his fate, to which we are inclined to attribute a more general significance." Mann can barely muster interest or empathy for his protagonist, but uses him to illustrate larger issues. This offended me, perhaps because it rendered illness, with which I was already intimately familiar, as less personal and real, as emblematic, a symbol for society's sickness. Castorp's mediocrity—and certainly a novel can focus powerfully on a mediocre main character—wasn't the problem for me; Mann's disdain and the imposition of his grandiose designs were. Of course, I understood that Mann's approach might be an exercise in irony, in satire, but that didn't alter things for me at all. He was messing with one of my sacred subjects, illness, just as I felt Pasternak was doing with his sappy handling of emotion, love, and poetry in *Doctor Zhivago*. The very things that shape *The Magic Mountain* as significant—its gravity, its subject, its tone and objectivity, its metaphoric intention—are at the heart of its failure for me.

Early in the novel, the deaths of Castorp's parents feel literary, not real, setting a pattern for how Mann presents illness itself. And whenever he seeks to be light and humorous, he sounds like the sort of person holding forth at a cocktail party who is far more entertained than his audience is by his wit. Everything that happens in the novel happens because Mann determines it, not because it flows from the characters' or the narrative's own lives. "A human being lives out not only his personal life as an individual, but also, consciously or subconsciously, the lives of his epoch and contemporaries." Well, to me, Mann neglected to give his characters those credible, individual personal lives.

Yet in 1996, when a paperback edition of *The Magic Mountain* appeared in a new translation, I bought a copy. This despite the familiar dismay I felt, standing in the bookstore aisle, just reading Mann's foreword, which takes six paragraphs to say that the story takes place before World War I, and includes this alarming, pompous statement about the novel's length and level of detail: "Unafraid of the odium of appearing too meticulous, we are much more inclined to the view that only thoroughness can be truly entertaining." After all, maybe my earlier problems were related to the translation, and besides, I had been sick again for nearly a decade with neurological damage caused by a viral attack. Maybe I was ready.

I wasn't ready in 1996, and I wasn't again in 2008, when I bought my last copy. This time, I failed to get past Castorp's first breakfast at the sanitarium. As with *Sophie's Choice* and *Doctor Zhivago*, *The Magic Mountain* is a novel that calls to some deep place in me as a reader, where desire and duty and need and personal experience all come together, repeatedly and at different times in my life, to override, at least initially, my aesthetic demands and expectations as a reader and writer. When I return to them, I return with a feeling of pressure, a yearning that outlives the conviction that a particular book will disappoint me.

Something else is going on with me and John Gardner's *The Sunlight Dialogues*. I knew Gardner, who was teaching medieval literature at Southern Illinois University when I arrived there in 1969 to study with Kinsella. This was before John Gardner became JOHN GARDNER. His first novel, *The Resurrection*, had been published to limited attention three years earlier, and the novels that were to make him famous hadn't yet appeared. On a shelf in his home office, Gardner had a series of black springback binders containing the completed manuscripts of *Grendel*, *The Sunlight Dialogues*, *Nickel Mountain*, and other books. Though none had been accepted, he continued writing new books, confident that publication would come.

That confidence was probably the most important thing I learned from Gardner. Well, also how to drink martinis. His eventual success, which began with the 1971 publication of *Grendel*, felt personal to me, something essential that I'd been permitted to witness though we were not close, a vindication of the sort of faith I was struggling to find for myself as a writer after leaving graduate school in June 1972.

In January 1973, a few months after *The Sunlight Dialogues* came out, I returned to southern Illinois to visit Gardner and ask him to inscribe a copy of the novel. Then I tried to read it, getting about two-thirds of the way through, to chapter XIII, which contains as its epigraph a line of poetry from Thomas Kinsella ("I only know things seem and are not good").

The Sunlight Dialogues was never a story toward which I felt irresistibly lured, that drew me emotionally, personally, the way *Sophie's Choice*, *Doctor Zhivago*, or *The Magic Mountain* did. Its cluttered, sometimes cartoonish account of a small-town police chief and his mystical prisoner, of upstate New York family agony, moved too slowly and unconvincingly at the police procedural level it had chosen for itself. It was marred by overwriting, sentence after sentence festooned with similes and metaphors that add nothing, that build toward nothing, are often inapt, and thrust the author into the foreground: "He took a long, slow drag on his pipe, casting about like an old woman in an attic for the meaning." Or, on the same page, the description of a police car starting up "clean and precise as a young child's tooth." Occurring multiple times on nearly every page, the almost random figurative outbursts create a kind of noise that drowns out story and character. Similarly, the effort at enchantment, the intrusive mythologizing and complexifying and magic just get in my way as a reader, as do the repeated use of Jewishness as a marker of unpleasant qualities ("He talked a great deal, in a way that at times made you think of a childlike rabbi" or, on the next page, he "opened his hands like a Jewish tailor" as though a Jewish tailor opened his hands differently than a gentile tailor). *The Sunlight Dialogues* is also too distracted by talk talk talk, as even the main character, Chief Clumly, notes, in a speech typical for its own interrupted flow: "'I don't listen much,' he said. 'A lot of—' He searched his mind. 'Lot of talk.'"

Yet I've tried to read the novel once every decade since that first attempt. In 1982, after Gardner died, I picked up *The Sunlight Dialogues* as an act of mourning. In 1993 I took it to Germany on my honeymoon, having told Beverly how much Gardner's example, and his occasional encouraging letters, had meant to me. And three years ago, when it came out in a New Directions reprint, I tried again, feeling that in some sense I still somehow owed it to his place in my memory to finish and even admire the novel that's considered his masterpiece.

A similar sense of obligation has led me to read no more than two hundred pages of Saul Bellow's *Humboldt's Gift* four times since 1975. I know I'm never going to accept the preposterous strand of Bellow's plot involving Chicago gangster Rinaldo Cantabile. I'm never going to deal with all the babble about the Austrian philosopher Rudolf Steiner and the central impact of his work on protagonist Charlie Citrine. But Bellow's fiction has meant so much to me, particularly *Seize the Day*, *Henderson the Rain King*, and *Herzog*, all of which I read as an undergraduate and which helped form my sense of what a prose writer might do, particularly with language; and I was intrigued by Bellow's use of the poet Delmore Schwartz as a model for the character who gives *Humboldt's Gift* its title; and I was living and working in Illinois at the time this very Illinois novel appeared. Plus, a writer and critic I admire, Sven Birkerts, wrote in his book *Reading Life: Books for the Ages* that *Humboldt's Gift* is his favorite novel, that it fills him "with the greatest covetousness" and inspires him to emulation. When he thinks of it, he immediately wants to write. I really wanted to like *Humboldt's Gift*, four times so far, but I know I won't ever. It's the only Bellow novel I've failed to finish.

Though it takes place, like *Sophie's Choice*, at a time and near an area where I lived, I can't finish—can barely read a dozen pages of—Jay Cantor's 2003 novel, *Great Neck*, which I've bought three times already. I can't read more than fifty pages of James Jones's *From Here to Eternity*, despite the fact that it's his Big Book, despite having lived in southern Illinois where he too lived, despite being compelled by his life story and having enjoyed several of his novels. I've got a copy I bought two years ago after having given away two previous copies. Pat Conroy's *The Great Santini*? I'm 0–4, having just this week set aside the last copy I will ever purchase, having broken my previous record by getting through eighty-eight pages before being exhausted by the caricature of its protagonist, whose lack of feeling for anyone, whose soulless programmed responses, fail to sustain my interest fully enough to find out how his family and his character might grow. I'm also 0–4 with John Fowles's *The French Lieutenant's Woman* and William Goldman's *Boys and Girls Together*.

Loyalty, homage, repayment, or admiration for the author, despite being insufficient motivations for finishing a particular piece of work, are obviously powerful draws for me when I consider what to read. But they are lesser draws than the deep, abiding connection I feel for crucial elements in such novels as *Sophie's Choice*, *Doctor Zhivago*, or *The Magic Mountain*. My finding that these lasting, canonical novels are unreadable, for me, is clarifying about the nature of my literary taste, perhaps also about my flaws as a reader. But the fact that over nearly four decades I've reacted so strongly as to discard and then replace copies shows something else, I think. In the presence of certain material, whether subject matter or style or emphasis or structure, I read with a combination of eagerness and avidity, of need and hope, that defines aspects of my essential self. I'm a reader, I've discovered, for whom the stakes can be absurdly high, and who—however experienced and trained and knowledgeable—is vulnerable to almost inexplicable passions and responses to the books that get most deeply under my skin.

What's more, I still have room on the bottom shelf for a half dozen or so books. Maybe this time, if I buy it, I can get through *A Tale of Two Cities*, which I last deposited in the trash on a train in Italy.

6

The Top Shelf

On Books I Need Beside Me

In 1972, while insisting that he was the wrong person to do so, the British poet Philip Larkin wrote a brief foreword for an Antiquarian Book Fair's program. After all, he said, "I should never call myself a book lover, any more than a people lover: it all depends on what's inside them." He also denied being a book collector, or even knowing how many books he owned. But Larkin did allow that he was a compulsive reader, "and this has meant that books have crept in somehow." So while he did not *love* or *collect* books he did need to *have* books. Many books, and always more books. "Only the other day," he wrote, "I found myself eyeing a patch of wall in my flat and thinking I could get more shelves in there."

More shelves! This is an attitude I can relate to, having crammed the tiny round house Beverly and I used to live in with so many straight-cornered bookshelves that I broke toes five times in fourteen years just trying to get into and out of my writing space. In our current, larger, and more rectilinear home, every room teems with bookshelves. The 137.5-square-foot bedroom where I write contains eight bookcases of varying shapes and sizes totaling 114 square feet of shelves. In our living room, the previous owner left a prodigious system of built-in, floor-to-ceiling shelves that made me giddy when I first saw them.

Like Larkin, I'm not a book collector, though I'll admit to having twenty-seven foreign and five American editions of my daughter's best-selling *The Immortal Life of Henrietta Lacks* in a glass-fronted bookcase opposite my writing desk. While not an indiscriminate book lover, either, the percentages show that I clearly share Larkin's need for books. And I can relate to his organizational approach. He had, he said, designated locations for specific types of books. Novels and detective stories were kept in his bedroom, "the higher forms of literature" and works about jazz were in his sitting room, titles "picked from a bad bunch on a station bookstall" and intended "to speed the parting guest" were in his hall. Shelved in the place of honor, "within reach of my working chair" and just to its left, Larkin kept books by twelve poets: "Hardy, Wordsworth, Christina Rossetti, Hopkins, Sassoon, Edward Thomas, Barnes, Praed, Betjeman, Whitman, Frost and Owen."

It's a revealing and not too surprising list, providing a gateway into thinking about Larkin's work. His to-hand poets are typically formal, traditional, plain spoken, direct, restrained, observant, often focused on disappointment or pain or loss. Excluding the flamboyant Whitman, the now-obscure nineteenth-century rural clergyman and dialect poet William Barnes (1801–86), and the even more obscure nineteenth-century politician and humorist Winthrop Mackworth Praed (1802–39), they're poets you would expect Larkin to have admired, to have turned to for refreshment and example as he worked. They're there, he says, "as exemplars."

I understand the need to keep such work close. It comes not only from the desire to reread or study or gain inspiration, but—at least for me—also from a talismanic impulse. So I too have a group of essential poets within reach of my working chair and just to its left. Not only within reach, but within view, so I can see them at a glance there on the top shelf of a small desktop bookcase. There's something more than admiration involved, something more intimate and emotionally urgent, a deeper connectedness.

My top shelf houses a never-changing core group of six poets: Frost, Eliot, Bishop, Stevens, Dylan Thomas, and Larkin himself. There's also Thomas Kinsella, the Irish poet with whom I studied and have remained friends for forty-four years, represented by both his *Collected Poems* and a two-CD compilation of his recorded readings, so I can hear his voice again. And there are other poets who rotate on or off the shelf, space currently occupied by Roethke, Williams, Lowell, Sexton, and Kinsella's Irish contemporary John Montague.

As I look over there now, and type the poets' names, it is difficult to keep my hands from leaving the keyboard to take down the Thomas. In three weeks, Beverly and I are going to Wales so we can visit some of the places he wrote about, and it'd be lovely right now to reread "Fern Hill." And wait, I want to check my recollection that Philip Larkin, long before admitting that he did fill his home with books, also wrote a poem in which he said that "books are a load of crap."

§

Nothing about my life until the age of twenty suggests that I would be a person who loved and wrote poetry. Who required it. My father, a citywide track champion whose dreams of Olympic competition failed to materialize, graduated from high school in 1926 and worked most of the rest of his thirty-five years, fifteen hours a day, in his Red Hook chicken market. My mother, who dropped out of school after ninth grade—also in 1926—was an aspiring chanteuse whose brief career ended after a fifteen-minute radio show aired on WBNX in the Bronx. The Melody Girl of the Air then found temporary work painting mannequins for theatrical costume designers until marrying my father in 1938. Trapped together in a small apartment or in the upstairs rooms of a rented house, they were disappointed in the way their lives had turned out, furious with each other and with their two children, seen as daily reminders of all they'd lost. Their mutual rage seethed between eruptions and required steady monitoring.

I grew up in a home where books were living room decor, their cream-and-red cloth bindings neatly lined up on one shelf among the bric-a-brac and plastic plants. No one read them; no one was allowed to touch them lest the covers be dirtied or misaligned. There were Balzac, Dumas, Flaubert, Maupassant, Zola—names my mother loved to pronounce with elaborately elongated first syllables. I can't recall my parents or brother reading a book. My father did read the newspaper when he got home at night, silent in his easy chair with a box of butterscotch cremes before him on the coffee table, and went to bed early so he'd be awake to open his market at dawn. I don't recall ever being in a bookstore until I went to college.

I had a few Hardy Boys volumes and Classics Illustrated comics, but was at best a haphazard and very occasional reader who seldom turned to books. My imaginative world was focused on playing with baseball cards or conducting two- or three-hour sessions of dice-baseball games during which I filled a notebook with extensive records of each player's performances. In this place of emotional chaos I tried to surround myself with order, with structure. Or I tried to be gone. I was active, playing ball in all seasons and in any league I could find, joining a youth group at the synagogue or a service organization at school, finding reasons to be at home as rarely as possible. When I was old enough, I got after-school and weekend jobs, busing tables, filing brochures at a travel agency, working as a butcher's apprentice, selling produce in a supermarket, cooking hamburgers at a beachfront snack bar, parking cars at beach clubs, mowing lawns.

Most of the books I remember reading as an adolescent had some connection with sports: *The Long Season* and *Pennant Race*, major league pitcher Jim Brosnan's memoirs of the 1959 and 1961 baseball seasons; Joe Garagiola's 1960 reminiscence, *Baseball Is a Funny Game*; Jimmy Breslin's 1963 account of the hapless New York Mets and their first season in existence the year before, *Can't Anybody Here Play This Game?*; biographies of Jackie Robinson or Mickey Mantle and sappy Young Adult baseball novels by John R. Tunis or Joe Archibald with the word *Kid* in their titles; Alan Sillitoe's 1959 novella, *The Loneliness of the Long Distance Runner*. I used the library, which was located near the town's railroad station on the way home from school, as a place where I could justifiably spend some time and delay my arrival home. I tended to take out the same books over and over.

I have no memory of reading poetry or being affected by hearing it until an afternoon in the spring of 1962, a few months after my father had died. I was nearing fifteen, a ninth-grader, when my English teacher read aloud A. E. Housman's "To an Athlete Dying Young," about the early death of a champion runner ("The time you won your town the race / We chaired you through the market-place"). As she asked questions afterward, I remember feeling thunderstruck, silenced, unable to move a muscle. Normally, I'd have found a way to tell about my father's exploits as an athlete, a runner like the young man suddenly dead in the poem. When class ended I couldn't get out of my seat. It felt as though Housman had reached someplace so far inside me that I hadn't known until then it was there. Nor had I known or had words to express quite what I thought or felt about my father's death, other than shock at its suddenness and finality, fear over what would happen to us without him, and anger at him for leaving me with my mother. But Housman seemed to know, specifically and personally, how harrowing it had been to see my father in his coffin, the terror of his eyelids sealed against me, "eyes the shady night has shut." He knew I couldn't forget the moment when the coffin was lowered, when I had to throw dirt on the coffin, heard it strike the wood above my father's face, and imagined him in there where "earth has stopped the ears." For all his speed in life, like the athlete in the poem my father was suddenly "Townsman of a stiller town." The contrast of swiftness and stillness, which I hadn't thought about before, seemed unbearable. But it also gave me a way to think about what I couldn't forget.

I was hardly the first adolescent to be bowled over by Housman's mix of romanticism, yearning, and loss, undone by the solemn tetrameters and heavy rhymes. But I did feel, right then in Mrs. Beckman's English class, as though Housman's poem were somehow mine, had spoken to and for me, had presented the eulogy I hadn't be able to say for my father. I've heard the poem spoken several more times since 1962—by Jim McKay, the great sportscaster, after Israeli athletes were murdered by terrorists during the 1972 Munich Olympics; by Meryl Streep, as Karen Blixen/Isak Dinesen in the film *Out of Africa*, after the death of her lover, Denys Finch Hatton—and it still triggers the same intense reaction, as though the particular sense of loss and shock were a dormant virus in my body being reactivated by exposure to Housman's words.

ⓢ

Despite—or perhaps because of—its impact, "To an Athlete Dying Young" didn't immediately alter my reading habits. Beyond what was required in school, poetry still had no place in my life. Why choose to read stuff that had such power to hurt? I did read a novel that was not about sports, John Le Carré's *The Spy Who Came In from the Cold*, since my aunt gave me a copy for my seventeenth birthday.

After graduating from high school, my primary motives for going to college were to get away from home and avoid being drafted. I had no sense of what I wanted to do or study or be. Maybe I would be a physical therapist or a chef, professions for which I had no more qualifications or calling than for any other. Maybe I could become an actor, since I had portrayed A-Rab in *West Side Story* during summer camp when I was fifteen. I did hope to play baseball for whatever college I went to.

It was the baseball fantasy that led me where I needed to go, because the only way I had a remote chance of playing college baseball was by attending a small, academically oriented school. With that in mind, and considering my mother's edict that I had to stay within 250 miles of home, and a transcript showing my best subjects were the nonsciences, my high school guidance counselor suggested that I apply to a pair of liberal arts schools whose admissions officers she'd recently spoken to: Colgate University and Franklin and Marshall College. I visited Colgate, in upstate New York, on a day when the temperature was twenty-six below zero. So I chose Franklin and Marshall, an all-male college in Lancaster, Pennsylvania, which I hadn't seen in person until the September afternoon when I moved into the dormitory. The decision that altered my life was based on nothing more substantial than who had been in contact with a guidance counselor I'd never known before entering her office, and the harsh weather in Hamilton, New York, on a winter day in early 1965.

At Franklin and Marshall, in another instance of serendipity, I was hired to be the reader for a blind professor, Dr. Robert Russell, who happened to be the chairman of the English Department. This assignment kept me around department activity, allowed friendships to develop with faculty members, made me feel involved with literature. It also began turning me into a serious reader as I tape-recorded novels, stories, and most often poems, including all the selections of Victorian era writers from *The Norton Anthology of English Literature*, a task that might have destroyed poetry for me forever but instead felt like some kind of grand initiation. To do the job properly required more than just a quick, flat recital that thumped along the metrical track. I needed a deeper engagement with the words and lines, an immersion in the poem's voice, its form's inner workings. I remember the skin-prickling excitement I felt, closed off in Russell's storage room with his reel-to-reel tape recorder and the massive textbook open before me, as I read Robert Browning's twelve-line poem of desire, "Meeting at Night." It might have been published in 1845 but it felt utterly NOW, the voice urgent and immediate and believable as the speaker brought his boat to land, leaped out on shore, and ran to the farmhouse where his beloved waited: "A tap at the pane, the quick sharp scratch / And blue spurt of a lighted match, / And a voice less loud, through its joys and fears, / Than the two hearts beating each to each."

This was astounding to me, more honest and open than Housman, real, emotional, barely-but-surely under control, and I loved it. I looked forward to coming to work, began putting in extra hours, took more and more English courses as electives, attended plays put on by the college's Green Room Theatre. Over the summers and on my own initiative I read Melville, Lawrence, Conrad—writers I'd been introduced to in classes. At the start of my junior year, I was officially an English major, Russell was my academic advisor, I'd auditioned for and been cast as Pompey in the Green Room's production of *Measure for Measure*, and I was no longer thinking about being a baseball player. Which was fortunate, because, near the close of a thoroughly mediocre freshman season, I'd sustained a shoulder injury that ended my playing days.

When I was asked by my family what I intended to do with a degree in English, the best answer I could offer was "get another one." I assumed I would complete an M.A. and Ph.D. and go on to teach, like the professors I'd come to admire and with whom I'd spent so much time. It was not that I particularly wanted to teach, or do research on a writer or specialize in an era—none of which I ended up doing. I just knew I'd become a person who loved to read, to think and talk about writing, and especially to speak written words—poems, prose, parts in plays—out loud. This act, this transference of words on a page to speech with the full engagement of my body and mind, satisfied something I didn't fully understand about myself.

☙

In the spring of 1969, as my final undergraduate semester began, I took a poetry writing class taught by Sanford Pinsker. He'd been hired the year before, after completing his doctorate at the University of Washington, where he'd gone in part to study with Theodore Roethke. But Roethke had died a month before Pinsker arrived in Seattle. So he ended up working with Roethke's colleague David Wagoner, hearing Roethke stories, and benefiting from fresh memories of Roethke's ideas about conveying emotional depth and immediacy, about rhythm and energy, formal tension over control of powerful feeling. He began reading the Confessional poets emerging in the mid-1960s—Berryman, Lowell, Sexton, Snodgrass—and I remember borrowing his copy of M. L. Rosenthal's 1967 study, *The New Poets*, and avidly reading its chapter on them. Near the book's end, I discovered excerpts from the work of someone I'd never heard of, Thomas Kinsella, who would soon come to mean so much to me.

Pinsker wrote poems and published them in magazines, but was also establishing himself as a critic of contemporary fiction, particularly Jewish fiction. This was his first writing class as a teacher, and my only writing class as a student. Pinsker was twenty-seven, fresh from being saturated in exactly the sort of poetry I most needed to know about, as enthusiastic about conveying a love and commitment to poetry as about teaching craft. It was the perfect moment for me to receive such instruction.

Although there were formal writing assignments or exercises, the class's emphasis was on close reading of poems from an anthology. Not only do I remember the book, I still have my copy, barely held together with old Scotch tape, pages highlighted and littered with notes. The binding is cracked in several places so that it lies flat when opened to Roethke's "The Lost Son," beside which I've exclaimed over and over, in green ink, the word "sounds!, sounds!"; or W. D. Snodgrass's "Heart's Needle, vi," where I've underlined and bracketed and starred the poet's comment "I shall have to investigate the objects and events of my personal life"; or Lowell's "The Quaker Graveyard in Nantucket," where I've blurted that "contemplation is the only means to salvation"; or Auden's "In Memory of W. B. Yeats," where I've repeated in the margins—IN ALL CAPS—that poetry "survives in the valley of its saying."

Reading Modern Poetry: A Critical Anthology, edited by Paul Engle and Warren Carrier, was a 1955 publication revised in 1968, the year before I bought it. Containing a generous selection of modern and contemporary poems arranged by increasing difficulty of reading, it also incorporated thorough analyses or commentaries—many written by the poets themselves—on several poems. It seemed as though these commentaries were addressed directly to me, as when Allen Tate wrote of the poet being in "a world that allows him but little certainty" or when Paul Engle said a poem could "become the live sound of a man talking intensely."

This book was where I encountered the poets who would remain touchstones for me and come to occupy my top shelf. The text of Stevens's "Sunday Morning," read and reread numerous times that spring, is so densely annotated that many lines are unreadable. "So sensual!" I wrote. And beside the final line, in which undulating pigeons sink "downward to darkness, on extended wings," there is just "Oh!" I can almost feel myself there, as a twenty-one-year-old, fully opening up to poetry for the first time. Underneath Elizabeth

Bishop's simple and clear lines in "The Map," I—the young man raised in an island home that threatened to drown us all in fury— have drawn a wavy pair of squiggles beneath the innocent-sounding lines "Along the fine tan sandy shelf / is the land tugging at the sea from under?"

Reading Modern Poetry is also where I found, in a comment by William Stafford about the writing of "Traveling through the Dark," a lasting justification for my urge to reexamine and write about dark childhood events that obsessed me: "an experience unfolds the depth any experience may conceal till it is touched and sprung into its poem. . . . Writing the poem becomes a process of discovering what elements contribute to the distinction of the event." Poetry would become an act of discovery for me, a way to make sense of experiences I could not escape.

It is also where I found that T. S. Eliot's "The Love Song of J. Alfred Prufrock," like so many other poems I had explicated in my Introduction to Poetry or Major British Writers courses, was not primarily a puzzle to decode but a moving and musical expression of emotion. I loved the way Eliot led me through Prufrock's physical and emotional wanderings as the long poem moved toward its devastating end, when thoughts of a walk upon the beach led him to say, "I have heard the mermaids singing, each to each. // I do not think that they will sing for me." The lines themselves held such loneliness, and when I noticed that Eliot had placed "I do not think that they will sing for me" as its own separate stanza, I registered the power of formal control at work.

Near the middle of the semester, Pinsker invited a young poet from New York to come down to Lancaster for a reading. He'd liked a poem of hers published in *New American Review*, and knew she'd just published a debut collection titled *Firstborn*. Louise Glück declined to do a reading, but agreed to visit the writing class. She was twenty-five, only four years older than we were, and looked haunted as she glowered from the cover of her book, body turned away but dark eyes cast back toward us, taking our measure, asserting distance, offering a testy welcome. It was a pose that suggested to me that the poetry she was offering came with some risk for both the poet and reader: *Are you ready for this?* it seemed to ask. *And am I?* I found it exciting to read her poems in preparation for the class. These early poems were, as critic William Logan has noted, "disconcerting, morbid," and "heavily marked by the influence of Sylvia Plath." In "Cottonmouth Country," she wrote about how "Death wooed us" and about "leaving a skin there" in the murky, sultry landscape of the southeastern shore. The poems combined anger with terrible vulnerability, a mix that I connected to, and they expressed a sense that those closest to us—our family, our friends, our lovers—were the most dangerous to us. Given my own tendency toward vigilance in such relationships, I knew what it meant when, in "The Wound," Glück said that she had "gone careful" while at her most intimate with someone. This was highly charged material dealt with in straightforward terms, but in language that managed to remain lyrical. A few of the poems, like "Bridal Piece," referred to the same south shore Long Island setting where I too had lived. The subject matter and the tone of her poems felt to me like an invitation, or a granting of permission—this was the way I must write, the opposite of impersonal, allusive, intellectual. Glück's poems were also "seductive" and taut, Logan wrote, "reduced to slivers of glass." Formally precise, often spoken by characters other than the poet, they showed me strategies for achieving a liberating distance within the enclosed dimension of form.

In class, she tolerated our comments and questions, read us a new poem, soon to appear in *New American Review* and subsequently, in 1975, in her second collection, *The House on Marshland.* It was the first time I had heard a poet—other than my classmates or Pinsker—read his or her work. In this instance, giving voice to such intense personal feelings through a poem spoken by a persona—by the fairy-tale heroine Gretel in the aftermath of having pushed the witch into the oven—Glück was performing and confessing at the same time, and I was mesmerized both by her and by the poem itself. "This is the world we wanted," she said, holding back the drama, letting the short sentence echo, dealing with her conflicting and nearly over-whelming emotions. "All who would have seen us dead / are dead."

If Louise Glück unintentionally granted me permission to be a poet, Anne Sexton clarified the terms. Pinsker had seen how Glück's visit had affected me and, a few weeks later, invited me along to hear Sexton read at Hood College, in Frederick, Maryland. Hood was an all-female school and we were the only males in the full audience, adding to the intensity, singularity, and strangeness of the experi-ence. By the time we arrived, I'd read all four books Sexton had published by then, including the new one, *Love Poems*, which came out only two months earlier, and I was hooked. Like Robert Lowell, with whom she'd studied at Boston University, Sexton undertook the delicate balancing of wild feeling and poetic restriction. But she seemed to me to write of even more extreme states, under greater pressure of emotion, and from a more volatile combination of inner and outer trauma. The poems' stability was not always assured. Their subjects—illness, family, love, the act of writing—were explored at their most threatening, and she made them sound at once essential and dangerous. Her best poems tended to rattle and rage in their confines, threatening their own very existence. The speakers some-times reminded me of my mother at her most crazed and desperate, then sometimes reminded me of myself trying to hold things together under the onslaught of madness around me. I read, and could not believe that someone other than I had written "The Black Art," which ended:

Never loving ourselves,
hating even our shoes and our hats,
we love each other, *precious, precious.*
Our hands are light blue and gentle.
Our eyes are full of terrible confessions.

Sexton, as she often did, began her reading with the poem "Her Kind." According to her biographer, Diane Wood Middlebrook, Sexton did this to show audiences "what kind of woman she was, and what kind of poet. . . . It was the way Sexton stepped from person to persona." But then, partway through the twenty-one-line poem, she began to cry, which tended to blur the distinction between person and persona, and underscore the way Sexton's poetry teetered between self-exploration and self-display. I remember realizing, in this fraught moment, that the poetry I was drawn to reading was poetry that drew little distinction between body and spirit, feeling and reason. I could hardly take my eyes off Sexton's hands, trembling as she turned pages, then balling into fists as she read.

Near the end of her reading, I heard a whisper and looked over at Pinsker sitting beside me. He was silent, looking at the ceiling with his eyes closed, mouth drawn tight, arms folded across his chest. It was the position of deep concentration that I recognized from class, and I knew he hadn't been the whisperer. Then it came again, and I almost vaulted from my seat. It was my own inner voice, the voice in my head, but somehow different too, calmer than usual, as though exerting patience until certain it had my attention. I took out a pen, turned over the flyer that announced Sexton's reading, and wrote the opening lines of what would become, more than a year later, the first poem I recognized as being in my own voice. *He parted the doors at four. / By eight the sawdusted floors / were patched with clots of feathers / and blood.*

When I looked up at Sexton again, and my mind returned to the room, she was saying the final lines of "Unknown Girl in the

Maternity Ward" in a voice almost shocking in its tenderness: "I choose / your only way, my small inheritor / and hand you off, trembling the selves we lose."

After the reading, Pinsker and I joined Sexton and some of the audience for an informal question-and-answer session in a smaller, more intimate room. I stood to her left and just behind her line of sight, knowing I should just listen and unable anyway to frame the question I wanted to ask. I took a deep breath, then felt Pinsker's comforting hand on my shoulder.

§

It's strange to recognize that almost all of my poetry-reading exemplars were identified during those thirteen weeks in the spring of 1969, in Pinsker's class. The poets who shaped me as reader and writer then have remained the poets I need beside me now. I know more of their work, and more of their lives, and that immersion has only deepened my appreciation. There are also many others, read and reread over the last forty-four years, whose work is important to me and who occasionally rotate onto the top shelf so I can engage with it again: Donald Hall, Seamus Heaney, Donald Justice, Maxine Kumin, Stanley Kunitz, Gibbons Ruark, Louis Simpson, Ron Slate, W. D. Snodgrass, Ellen Bryant Voigt, Richard Wilbur. And there are individual poems by these and others that I turn to. But my top shelf, in the fifteen homes I've lived in since leaving Lancaster in 1969, has had a consistent core of occupants.

Last month, I spoke with Sanford Pinsker for an hour. He's retired, living in Florida, and while he remembers hearing Anne Sexton read several times, doesn't recall our trip to Hood College. What he does remember is a series of phone calls from me in the years after I graduated, as I studied for a year with Thomas Kinsella, then worked for seventeen years in the field of public policy before becoming disabled in 1988. In those phone calls, he says, I would talk about the poetry I was reading, or we'd discuss my poems, and he understood how important poetry still was to me, even though I was working with budgets and governments.

"The roots were there," he said, "a deep love of poetry that deepened instead of going away."

Which gave me the opportunity I hadn't known I was waiting for. "You should know, Sandy. You're the one who planted those roots."

Pinsker's class, and its timing in my life, could not have been better for me. Without realizing it, I'd been moving closer to a life in poetry. I was in the right place when a young teacher offered his first writing class, a young poet agreed to visit that class, and a prize-winning poet overcame the forces that would lead to her suicide five years later and was able to put on a performance that would liberate me to begin writing in my own voice. "Today is made of yesterday, each time I steal / toward rites I do not know," Sexton wrote in "The Lost Ingredient." I believe that this is precisely what is permitted to me by having the work of Frost, Eliot, Bishop, Stevens, Thomas, Larkin, Roethke, or Sexton herself so close. They make my work possible.

7

SOMETHING TO MARVEL AT

Discovering Jules Verne at Sixty

As Beverly and I walked down the sodden creekside trail, sounds of traffic from Interstate 84 behind us gradually turned into the sound of Latourell Falls ahead of us. The transition was complete when the creek bent east to open a sudden view of the falls cascading down the north side of Pepper Mountain. We stopped to watch its 250-foot plunge. Though only thirty miles east of Portland, in the Columbia River Gorge, the spot felt like a passageway into another world.

Deeper in the woods, the morning darkened and chilled. But like an echo of sunlight, otherworldly bright yellow lichen flourished on the basalt column beside the falls. Ice lingered here and there on exposed rock as though time moved differently here. Provided we didn't think about the neatly carved directional signs marking the trail, the weathered benches, a wooden bridge across Latourell Creek, or swarms of tourists chattering and listening to iPods, the scene was almost prehistoric: a damp, densely firred canyon filled with reverberation from the falls, strange hues all around, deadfall hosting swarms of lush life, birds darting through shafts of mist. From just the right perspective, it was a vision of the truly marvelous, a teeming spot where the distant past thrived within the familiar present.

⟡

Trained as a geologist, a former master gardener, now an impressionist landscape painter, and avid birder, Beverly is at home in the natural world. Her knowledge and instinct allow her intimate connection to forms of the earth, an appreciation for cycles of growth and loss, a grasp of the history contained within the wild. She liked being there by the falls.

Brooklyn born, a city dweller until I married Beverly and lived for thirteen years with her in the woods of rural western Oregon, I remain much less in tune with nature. Engaged, an alert and attentive observer, I'm more edgy and wary, detached rather than comfortable. Also, my balance still compromised twenty years after the viral attack that had damaged my brain, I found the uneven footing beside Latourell Creek difficult, the ups and downs quickly tiring. But I followed as Beverly moved through the woods taking photographs, describing what rocks revealed, naming plants and trees.

Near the frothing pool where the falls crashed with full force, I found myself thinking that this was just the sort of place Jules Verne could have set a scene in his sixty-four-work series known as the *Extraordinary Journeys*. Strange, isolated, out of time, with the outsize power of nature on full display. But without, of course, the smart and beautiful woman. Or the disabled man.

A Verne novel's calm, masculine hero would be accompanied by a powerful male sidekick and a loyal assistant, as the harpoonist Ned Land and manservant Conseil accompanied Professor Aronnax onto Captain Nemo's submarine, the *Nautilus*, in *20,000 Leagues Under the Sea*; nephew Axel and guide Hans accompanied Professor Otto Lidenbrock into the volcano in *Journey to the Center of the Earth*;

servant Passepartout accompanied gentleman Phileas Fogg in *Around the World in 80 Days*; or the reporter Gideon Spilett, sailor Pencroff, and his courageous boy Harbert accompanied engineer Cyrus Smith and his servant Neb in *The Mysterious Island*. There might even be a male dog or monkey too, as in *The Mysterious Island*. Rather than a midday sightseeing destination just beyond a city's suburb, Latourell Falls would be located on an uncharted island or in some far-off outpost at the remote end or the deep core of the planet. And despite the pristine beauty, it would be plagued by threatening creatures and people with evil intentions. The man standing here, looking around, would be, like Cyrus Smith, "very learned, very practical." He would be "an unusually resourceful person," someone "ever ready for anything, competent in everything" as he explored the unknown, facing down every threat, making his own way. A man "of great mettle . . . a man of action." He would, in sum, be unlike me in every way. And any women would be back home, yearning for their men to return, not leading a limping, aging fellow thinking about stories of fictional adventure.

৯

Verne had been on my mind lately, though I'd never read any of his books. I'd seen the movies *20,000 Leagues Under the Sea* and *Around the World in 80 Days* more than fifty years ago, but all I remembered were a giant squid attack near the end of the former, and a fancy souvenir book I got when seeing the latter at Radio City Music Hall in 1956. Giant squid, that was Jules Verne to me. When Beverly and I ordered squid at a restaurant in Provence three summers earlier, and the dish consisted of a reeking rubbery white slab instead of the small fried rings we had anticipated, I'd set it aside after one taste, saying that it looked like something out of Jules Verne. To me, based on no direct encounters with the work, Verne was a writer of things monstrous, tales of the earth and its creatures run amok, a science fictiony/horror hack, a nineteenth-century Stephen King, whose work I also hadn't read.

But now I was reconsidering Verne. It began a few weeks earlier, when Beverly and I were talking about childhood movies that had made lasting impressions on us. I named 1954's *Seven Brides for Seven Brothers*, a schmaltzy musical-western-love-story I saw at age seven, fascinated by a world so alien to my own. I still know all its forgettable songs by heart. I also mentioned *The Defiant Ones*, from 1958, in which Sidney Poitier and Tony Curtis play escaped convicts chained together as they flee through the South. I saw it with my brother when I was eleven and he, at nineteen, was someone to whom I had often felt awkwardly shackled as we fled our parents' rages. Beverly talked about *Pollyanna*, from 1960, and how strongly she resonated with the Haley Mills character's positive outlook, the way it changed everybody's life for the better. She also named *Journey to the Center of the Earth*, which as a child had fascinated and frightened her, lured and repelled her, its scenes remaining vivid for nearly fifty years. She wondered if it was behind her collegiate desire to study geology.

Shortly after that conversation, we watched a new, made-for-television version of *Journey to the Center of the Earth*, starring Rick Schroder, Peter Fonda, and Victoria Pratt. It was set in 1870s Alaska rather than 1860s Iceland, and transformed Verne's story of a scientist's quest for discovering the earth's core into an abandoned woman's search for her missing husband. Throughout the program, Beverly pointed out the ways this travesty altered the original movie's narrative. She kept saying we should be sure to see the 1959 version she knew and loved, and that I'd missed altogether.

I went online to order a copy at Amazon.com and looked around at other material by Jules Verne. That was when it struck me: not only had I never read his work, I had never read Robert Louis Stevenson, James Fenimore Cooper, Arthur Conan Doyle, Jack London, H. G. Wells, Alexandre Dumas, none of the great authors of boyhood adventure classics. Never read *Gulliver's Travels, King Solomon's Mines, The Red Badge of Courage,* or *Robinson Crusoe* either.

One of the few classics I'd read outside of school was Mark Twain's *A Connecticut Yankee in King Arthur's Court,* given to me by a kindly man who came to our house to draw blood one summer when I was sick with mononucleosis. Those months, when I was eleven and sequestered in bed, would have been the perfect time to read Jules Verne, to escape my bedroom and journey to distant, exotic places, have thrilling escapades, be reminded that, as he wrote in *20,000 Leagues Under the Sea,* "hope is so strongly rooted in the heart of man!"

Despite bachelor's and master's degrees in English, I never caught up with those boyhood adventure books along the way. And over the last twenty years, despite frequently feeling the need to find in reading an escape from the confinement and limitations that accompany long-term illness, I had not thought of trying those boyhood adventure books. Why not start now, at sixty, with Jules Verne and his stories of escape to the middle of nowhere?

Beverly's enthusiasm for the movie version of *Journey to the Center of the Earth* also made me speculate about whether I'd been missing something essential in my reading, something similar to what had gripped her about the movie. The irresistible pull of traditional storytelling, the full absorption that comes with being enthralled by a fictional world. I wondered if Jules Verne could return that to me.

I was aware that my reading had undergone a steady shift away from fiction, and that I felt a desire for refreshment of my thirst for it. Going back to my reading diary, I saw that in the year 2000, I'd read 102 books, and 68 of them—exactly two-thirds—were fiction. The next year, I read 106 books, and 55 of them were fiction, so the percentage of my reading devoted to fiction had dropped to just over half. It was a trend that continued in a straight line throughout the first eight years of this century. By 2004, I was down to 43 percent fiction. Last year, of the 85 books I read, only 24 were fiction. Just 28 percent.

This had been an unplanned but sure alteration of my reading habits. I think that as I neared sixty, and completed the second decade of my illness, something changed about the spell novels cast for me. I was starting and abandoning novels, failing to sustain imaginative connection, and was turning toward literary biographies, narrative nonfiction, memoirs, cultural histories, reindulging my childhood passion for baseball books. Either something was missing in the fiction I was reading, or something had changed in me. I still had a substantial shelf of fiction, but was not drawn to it when the time came to select a new book. I was, though, still longing for the pleasure of direct, unadorned storytelling and character development. I just wasn't finding it in the contemporary fiction at hand. "The human mind," Jules Verne wrote in *20,000 Leagues Under the Sea*, "is always hankering after something to marvel at." Reading fiction, which had for so long satisfied that hankering in me, was not doing so anymore.

🌀

To tell his most compelling stories, and create his most convincing characters, Jules Verne relied on a simple recurring premise: isolate a small group of individuals and have them undergo fantastical adventures in an alien, dramatic, threat-filled natural setting. "A world apart," he called it in *20,000 Leagues Under the Sea*, where the limited cast must rely on fortitude, ingenuity, agility of spirit and body, and teamwork to survive extreme conditions. No drawing rooms, no domestic dramas, no offices in Jules Verne's best novels.

He worked variations on this fundamental setup, which in essence was the deserted island motif. In the case of my favorite Verne novel, *The Mysterious Island*, it was a literal unmapped, deserted South Seas island to which five balloon-borne escapees from a confederate prison camp in Richmond, Virginia, are blown during a long and ferocious storm. In the case of *20,000 Leagues Under the Sea*, it was a submarine, the *Nautilus*, equipped to be self-sustaining as it wandered beneath the oceans without a home port, its only contact with other humans hostile and warlike. A mobile, submerged island. *Journey to the Center of the Earth* was set primarily within the planet's vast underworld accessed from inside a volcano located in "barren landscape of Iceland at the edge of the world." A network of caverns and passages permitted the cut-off characters to wander through earth's hidden corescape without encountering other humans. In *Around the World in 80 Days*, Phileas Fogg and his manservant, Passepartout, embark on an intensely self-contained expedition that, while not literally stranding them in isolation, maintains them as a separate unit seeking to avoid any contact that might delay their progress toward circumnavigation of the globe in the specified number of days. They are a kind of traveling island. Or are, as Passepartout observes, "journeying in a dream" as they pursue their surreally insulated quest.

The premise alone didn't, of course, ensure success. Many of Verne's lesser tales made use of it too: the early novel, *The Adventures of Captain Hatteras*, involved the crew of a ship, the *Forward*, led from Liverpool by the doomed, monomaniacal John Hatteras on a demented journey in search of the North Pole. But Verne hadn't yet learned to incorporate his prodigious research into his fictional narrative, or to use dialogue as a means of propelling action rather than providing information, and the novel failed to sustain momentum. Similarly flawed by belabored scientific and geographical data, sketchy characterization, and patchwork plotting was the bare, undeveloped late novel, *Lighthouse at the End of the World*, in which a trio of men deployed to manage the new lighthouse on uninhabited Staten Island, near the South Pole, found themselves combating a gang of piratical malefactors.

While his desert island formula might be guaranteed to captivate boyhood readers, to work on a skeptical sixty-year-old man in a fiction-reading slump, it had to offer depth of character and believability of action. It had to offer more than the surface razzmatazz of scientific, natural, or geographical exotica. For me, what made Verne's work riveting—almost despite its sci-fi or adventure pyrotechnics—was its deft, convincing consideration of isolated characters under duress, thrown back on their essential selves in order to survive. I know this had something to do with my own situation as a reader, but I think it has attraction for a wide range of other readers as well, captivated by the basic confrontation of man and the most extreme conditions, most dire threats to integrity of mind, body, and soul. At his best, Verne also channeled into his provocative situations and settings a sense of his own loneliness and detachment, yearning for shared adventure and small group solidarity, wealth of scientific knowledge laced with concern over how science would be applied, and fantasies of escape. He took the time to explore personality, not just sketch figures as he told the rip-roaring tales of adventure that captivated his mind, and he avoided the lecture hall mode—the dispensation of information—that often had crippled his other narratives. Verne's achievement was to anchor the incredible in bedrock credibility of detail, the Romantic in straightforward naturalness, isolating characters under intense pressure and finding out what qualities sustained them.

⑨

Not a scientist, Verne taught himself enough science to ground his stories in the latest discoveries, speculate on what further discoveries might follow, and project how they might alter human behavior. He convinced himself that science offered answers to everything, as Cyrus Smith, hero of *The Mysterious Island*, explained: "I don't believe in chance, no more than I believe in earthly mysteries. There is a cause for every inexplicable event." Not a philosopher, Verne found his way to a few profound ontological insights that he was able to express in fictional action, or in his characters' thoughts, such as Professor Otto Lidenbrock's resonant existential message, given to his acrophobic nephew, Axel, as they prepared for their explorations in *Journey to the Center of the Earth*: "Look down carefully! We must take lessons in abysses." Not a world traveler, though he did spend eight days in America—his only journey outside Europe—and certainly not an explorer, Verne imagined credibly the most remarkable, state-of-the-art journeys to unsettled, distant places and brought them to vivid life, as with the Klondike of *The Golden Volcano*, a late novel published posthumously, or the meticulously detailed underwater landscape, the "wonderland" full of "liquid light" in *20,000 Leagues Under the Sea*. Not a man of action, he created a series of men of action wholly believable in their mix of ingenuity, bravery, conviction, and compulsion.

Verne's inner life, to judge from his finest fiction, was all about being other, going elsewhere, escaping from the life he was leading. Applying what he knew and imagined in ways that he couldn't manage in his daily life. It was about honoring in his writing the wildest of those imaginings, or, as he has the manservant Conseil, an otherwise carefully constrained character, explain in *20,000 Leagues Under the Sea*, "Don't reject the existence of something just because you have never heard of it." Willing himself out of the trap of himself, he found a kind of joyful freedom in the dream of fiction, the convincing creation of the marvelous. As Professor Lidenbrock said, facing almost certain death while trapped in the erupting core of a volcano, "As long as the heart beats, as long as the flesh pulsates, I can't admit that any creature endowed with willpower needs to be overwhelmed by despair." All this, the combination of learning and imagination, the escape that forces us deeper into the real, the journey outward and away that brings us further inward and home, the balance of individual and communal interests that enable us sometimes to meet extreme challenge, is what made Verne's best novels compelling for me.

That he managed to write four enduring novels at all was an act comparable to the staunch triumphs of his dogged, ingenious protagonists. Jules Verne was born in northwest France in 1828. His father was a lawyer from Nantes, his mother a well-educated Breton, and Verne grew up on manmade Feydeau Island, where the Loire River flows through Nantes, with a view of the harbor and sea.

He came by his lifelong fascinations early, simply by looking out the window or wandering the streets. According to William Butcher in *Jules Verne: The Definitive Biography* (2006), "Quayside ships literally overshadowed the front door" and young Verne could watch the tides bring in everything from sardine boats to lost porpoises. He "learned about nautical operations at an early age." Feydeau Island was a place where Jules Verne's sensibility was shaped by local tales of adventure in far-off locales, by images of water and ships and islands and floating cities, the allure of travel, exotic escapades, extraordinary voyages, escape. The urge to travel would, Butcher writes, become "the alpha and omega of Verne's writing and life." He read and was compelled by *The Swiss Family Robinson* and *Robinson Crusoe*, dreamed of being a castaway, even tried to stow away on an ocean-going vessel at the age of eleven. In tandem with this obsession over remote travel, an obsession never acted upon in real life, Verne encountered make-believe all around. Even the island he lived on was fabricated. "All the books he wrote," says Verne's great-grandson Jean on the A&E Television Network's *Biography* video, "it was the life he dreamed to have when he was a boy."

Seems like the ideal situation for a writer-in-the-making. But Verne's family wanted him—expected him—to become an attorney and join his father's practice. No rebel, Verne tried to comply. He moved to Paris, studied law, dabbled in commerce, attempted the civic life. But he found himself gravitating toward and coming to love the literary life instead. He attended salons and became close friends with both Alexandre Dumas the elder and Alexandre Dumas the younger. He met editors, publishers, and critics, met painters and musicians. Soon he began to write plays, several of which were performed. He also wrote short stories, a study of the Paris Salon exhibition of 1857, a study of Edgar Allan Poe, music criticism, then branched out into novel-writing. Verne's father disapproved, but eventually agreed to provide some support while his son struggled.

Verne also discovered a passion for study. He loved going to the library to research ideas, teaching himself as much as he could about the new developments in science that were changing the world around him. Evidence of man's ingenuity, and of relentlessness in its pursuit, fascinated Verne throughout his creative life. He admired it in others and sought to practice it in his writing. Butcher remarks on Verne's "remarkable capacity for sustained work," a quality that would enable him to write several books each year for more than forty years. In addition to showing us the romance of the imaginary journey—the incredible expedition—Verne "opened our eyes to the romance of science," as producer and screenwriter Gavin Scott says on the A&E *Biography* video.

After two apprentice novels, *Five Weeks in a Balloon* (1863) and *The Adventures of Captain Hatteras* (early 1864), things quickly came together for Verne as a fiction writer. Between late 1864 and 1875—between the ages of thirty-six and forty-seven—he published the four novels on which his literary achievement rests: *Journey to the Center of the Earth* (late 1864), *20,000 Leagues Under the Sea* (1870), *Around the World in 80 Days* (1873), and *The Mysterious Island* (1875). It was an impressive heyday, on a lesser scale of accomplishment but comparable to Thomas Hardy's sustained excellence between 1886 and 1895, when he wrote *The Mayor of Casterbridge*, *The Woodlanders*, *Tess of the d'Urbervilles*, and *Jude the Obscure*.

It was also an inconsistent heyday, unlike Hardy's, since Verne also published seven far lesser novels during those years. *From the Earth to the Moon*, for example, appearing in 1865, was remarkable for its predictions about space travel—including a satellite launch from southern Florida and a projected splashdown in the ocean—but was marred by a ham-handed satire of America, a lack of fully developed scenes, unconvincing characterization, and long disquisitions on the science of launch or flight that extensively interrupt the story's flow. It hardly seems conceived as a novel, but rather as a series of essays about planetary bodies and flight dynamics and ballistics and mathematics linked together by the barest outline of a narrative. Also published in this period were such long-forgotten novels as *Adventures of Half a Dozen Savants, The "Great Eastern,"* and *Journey to the Fur Country.*

Not just during Verne's eleven-year peak, but throughout his long career, his achievement was obscured by the great quantity of lesser work. During his lifetime, he published over fifty novels as well as books of short fiction and nonfiction. After his death, another ten books appeared, often in versions revised by his son, Michel. This astonishing productivity was, in part, due to Verne's own desire and capacity for work, but also to a contractual arrangement—almost inconceivable for a trained lawyer to have signed—which obligated him to at least two novels annually with meager compensation. So he was working for the paltry money as well as to satisfy his contract and his own drive. And, again like Thomas Hardy, he worked as an alternative to spending time with his mismatched wife. Verne's publisher, Jules Hetzel, also exerted powerful influence on the contents of his bestselling novelist's work, censoring political or romantic content, cultural observation, character traits, storyline.

But in his four best novels, Verne overcame these limitations, overcame as well his problems with incorporating research into the narrative line and his tendency toward despair when considering how human beings would mess up the glorious possibilities he envisioned for scientific advance. The novels read like sustained dreams, and Verne seemed to lose himself in the sheer joy of going away, imaginatively, to his various worlds apart.

Near the end of *20,000 Leagues Under the Sea*, Verne had its narrator, Professor Aronnax, speak for the author and his achievement when he told us, "I am a writer whose business it is to record things that appear impossible yet are incontestably real. This was not a dream. I saw and felt what I am describing." His stories work when their dream-like quality strikes the reader as utterly real, when their fundamental escapism seems like a passage to discovery. When, through fullness of characterization and directness of narrative, they sustain the spell cast by their inventiveness.

⑤

I read *Journey to the Center of the Earth* during a two-day February trip from Portland to Los Angeles, getting through most of it on the planes. As I read, I kept thinking how much Verne would have loved air travel (Portland to Los Angeles in two and a half hours!). He wouldn't have been as irritated as I was by the delays and cramped seating and bumpy ride, or the forty-degree temperature difference between northern Oregon and Southern California. And he wouldn't have spent his flight time reading a novel. He'd be doing research and conjuring adventures so that novel-readers might experience something to marvel at. So that we might be liberated from our over-familiarity with things of this world, and be made to see them, and thereby ourselves, freshly. If he couldn't talk his way into the cockpit, he'd be wandering the cabin to look out windows on both sides, front and back, studying the skies and ground, making calculations, distracted only by the information about airspeed and altitude and temperature on the computer screen in the seatback before him. In 1876, when Verne was forty-eight and had written several books about balloon travel, he finally took a brief flight in one himself, but otherwise his airborne journeys were limited to pure imagination, an imagination that envisioned airplanes, guided missiles, even the space satellite—though in *From the Earth to the Moon* the satellite is launched by a large cannon rather than a rocket—long before their actual invention.

After our return to Portland, Beverly and I finally watched the 1959 film version of *Journey to the Center of the Earth* that had made such an impression on Beverly. At first, all I could see were the ways in which Hollywood had changed Verne's story, from the characters' names (Sir Oliver Lindenbrook instead of Otto Lidenbrock, making him Scottish instead of German), relationships (transforming nephew Axel into the unrelated student Alec McEwan and, as played by Pat Boone, having him croon "A Red, Red Rose"), and motivations, to the plot that added a female to the exploration team, a pet duck named Gertrude, and a Swedish treasure-hunter kidnapping the heroes temporarily. But with Beverly's help, I got past my kvetching and began to enjoy the cinematic imagery—particularly the re-creation of Verne's imagined underground ocean and storm—that was the film's truest connection to its literary source. I also began to accept the characters, especially the resourceful and monomaniacal Lindenbrook, as played by James Mason, rather than comparing them to the original versions. I surrendered to the suspense of the journey despite knowing that all would end happily. So I got into the Jules Verne zone, learning to overlook the film's flaws and experience the combination of escape and discovery, fact and invention, possibility and preposterousness, that are so crucial to his work. After all, if Verne could write of a space launch propelled by a cannon in *From the Earth to the Moon*, why could director Henry Levin not have the characters in *Journey to the Center of the Earth* escape an erupting volcano by riding on the molten lava in a kind of asbestos teacup.

As I began working my way through nine Verne novels, and watching movie versions that wildly distorted four of them, I came to appreciate Verne's great gift for portraying mixed motives. He was a master of the paradoxical pull between loneliness and companionship, risk and security, the ties of home and the freedom of travel, capturing these tensions in moments of great resonance: Captain Nemo, sealing himself off from the world but treasuring the company of his small crew, shattered by their deaths and ritually honoring each with a sacred burial on the sea floor; Phileas Fogg risking his wager to rescue Passepartout, who had been captured by Indians after risking his life to save Fogg; the castaways of *The Mysterious Island* yearning for rescue even as they love the life created together on their island. At the end of that wonderful novel, the rescued group of survivors sets up a colony in Iowa so they can continue living the life apart together.

I also came to appreciate the ways in which Verne, on occasion, did cast the spell I had been looking for when reading fiction. In *The Mysterious Island* particularly, in much of *Journey to the Center of the Earth* and *20,000 Leagues Under the Sea*, and occasionally in *Around the World in 80 Days*, I found myself drawn back each time I put down the book, found myself immersed. I was unaware of the writer or the writing, maintaining imaginative connection to the characters and their story, marveling at the revelations of character and scene.

At the same time I was reading Verne, Beverly was painting a twelve-by-sixteen picture called *Latourell Creek in Fall*. It now hangs where we most often sit to read together. Inspired by our visit to Latourell Falls, and informed by the photographs Beverly had taken while we were there, her painting is an impressionistic response, full of broken forms, shifting patterns, and vivid autumn colors that suggest both the energy and fleeting light within the scene. Exciting, exotic, a remote landscape, it also conveys a feeling of calm in the presence of such force, and a deep familiarity with the hidden underlying geological structures. It captures the place, but also captures Beverly's response to it. I easily lose myself in it, as I lose myself in reading Verne, and it reminds me of the impetus to begin reading Jules Verne at age sixty, my desire for a fresh appreciation of something I had been missing, the marvel of original storytelling.

Part Three

A SPINNING WORLD

The ear that hears wind chatter in cedar
woods listens also to the earth curve
beneath your feet. It holds you in place
as you move through a spinning world.

Floyd Skloot,

from "Balance"

8

THE SIDE EFFECT
OF SIDE EFFECTS

On August 8, 1990, I had "a neurological event." I know it was August 8 because the only thing I was able to say for several hours was *How could it be August 8?* I know it was 1990 because I was about to participate in the clinical field trial of a new drug that might be able to treat the viral illness I'd contracted twenty months earlier, targeting my brain and leaving me so neurologically shredded I was judged totally disabled by the Social Security Administration and my skeptical insurance company. To qualify for inclusion in the drug trial, I had to have a spinal tap. It didn't matter that I had one a year earlier for diagnostic purposes. Results of medical research have to be standardized, and each subject in the drug trial had to undergo procedures analyzed by the same lab in the same way at the same time.

Either the tap, itself a breach of cerebrospinal integrity, or a leak of spinal fluid from the site where the tap occurred, or the resulting dehydration despite all the water I dutifully drank, or a further worsening of neurological damage caused by a reactivation of the virus we were hoping to counteract or of my immune system after the introduction of a needle into my body, or some other unknown trigger had caused me to wake up on the morning of August 8, 1990, unable to figure out where I was in time or space, what was happening, or what I could do to make sense of it. Apparently, I found the morning newspaper and saw the date. Then I called my former wife, said *how could it be August 8?* over and over, in response to each comment or question, hung up, and went back to bed until the doorbell rang. I opened the door, naked, and greeted the woman—our new realtor, who lived down the street and had been called to help by my former wife—by saying *how could it be August 8?* She looked at my eyes, her gaze never drifting, told me to get dressed, and waited on the porch.

I woke up on a gurney in the emergency room at Oregon Health Sciences University, not far from where I'd had the spinal tap. My daughter was there, was not, was. My doctor came in, wiggled the IV line rehydrating my system, nodded as he spoke. It was not a stroke. It was not a tumor. It was a neurological event. These things happen. Not his fault. I will be all right. I nodded back. Of course of course. A horse is a horse of course of course. I will be all right. What, exactly, does he mean by all right? When? I can't go home until I can pee.

I was in the hospital, so I was no longer lost in space. My daughter looked the same age I remembered her being before, a month shy of eighteen, so I was no longer lost in time. Or not too lost. Because I still had no idea how it could be August 8. Temporal uncertainty: another way of saying where I was. Temporal lobe: another way of saying where my brain lesions were. Temporal bone: another way of saying where my skull was about to explode.

Just over eight months later, the drug trial was suspended. No one got better. A lot of us, including me, got worse. But for the time being, I still had hope, had faith, that some drug or procedure or therapy might fix me.

I took a prescription drug that left me absolutely convinced a gust of wind was the reincarnation of Vladimir Nabokov. He was chasing butterflies through a meadow that didn't exist in the woods behind our house. The odd thing was that he moved in waltz time when the music I heard was definitely samba.

I'd been seeing him for a few days, ever since I started taking the drug, but I could usually convince myself he was nothing but a trick of light. Not now, though, not anymore. Because just above the crest of the hill, and just out of Nabokov's reach, a pair of Spring Azure butterflies danced on air as they sang Reel 2 Real's 1994 hit "I Like to Move It" with Russian accents.

When at my doctor's suggestion we adjusted the dosage, I really missed Nabokov for a few days. He'd seemed uncharacteristically happy there in the woods, wandering through morning mist with his net raised, looking more like an elk than a man. A ghost. I think it was the sense of being disembodied that drew me to him, made me feel we were in the moment together. Both of us in a realm beyond the corporeal. Being outside my body seemed like a good thing then.

I took a prescription drug that speckled my skin like rust on a hollyhock. I was away from home at the time, in Baltimore, and it was August, over a hundred degrees, heavy with humidity, so I thought the rash was prickly heat.

The problem with that diagnosis was that the rash didn't resemble prickly heat's red millet seed eruptions, was not particularly prickly, and covered nearly my whole body. So then I thought it was shingles, since I'd caught the chicken pox a year earlier, the last time I was in Baltimore, and maybe now it had reactivated as shingles. Happens. The problem with that diagnosis was that the rash didn't resemble shingles' crusty blisters, or hurt much.

The rash didn't come off when I showered, or after I slept, or when I forced myself not to look at it for three hours straight, or when I took a walk, or when I drank red wine. I needed a diagnosis. Which I got when I called my dermatologist and she asked if I'd started a new drug recently. The rash went away when I stopped taking the new drug. At which point the doctor who had prescribed it suggested that I start taking it again because how could we know for sure that the drug made me break out in the rash. No.

I took a drug that made me faint when I peed in the middle of the night. Another made me pee vivid shades of saffron, coral, and cantaloupe. And another made me feel like I was at the halfway point of a hundred-meter dash and another made me so anxious I had to take another drug to calm down. None of these drugs were meant to cure the thing that was really wrong with me, the neurological damage. Something like that, I came to understand, doesn't get cured. The acute phase runs its course and leaves behind its aftermath. Aftermaths were what I was working on. Pain, sleep disturbance, neurotransmission problems, failures of mitochondrial energy production.

I took a drug that made me stink. I smelled so foul that people recoiled when I entered a room. My arrival at a friend's office knocked another visitor back into the chair she'd just risen from. At the meat counter in Safeway, shoppers nearby would frown and reject the packages they were looking at, convinced of spoilage. My odor was an intense combination of garlic, sweaty socks, burnt plant matter, and organic rot. Later, Beverly referred to it as *Eau de Stinky*. I couldn't smell it myself. I'd been warned, I could see its impact, but my stench was only an abstraction to me. I just felt thirsty all the time, and the taste in my mouth was like Skookum oysters about a week beyond their sell-by date. There's a significant difference between hearing that a drug has the side effects of bad breath and body odor and seeing those effects overwhelm any space I entered.

I was taking this drug as an experiment. It had been used successfully on horses with sore muscles. It had been used successfully on humans in the United States for a disease I didn't have, interstitial cystitis. In the later half of the twentieth century, it had been used successfully in the Soviet Union for rheumatic diseases, which I also didn't have. It reduced abdominal adhesions in rats, neither of which were my problems.

Patients with pain rubbed it on the areas that hurt. For certain diseases, patients drank it. For other diseases, patients received intravenous infusions. It was administered to me, over the course of three months, by all means available. I drank it daily, rubbed it here and there three times a day or more if pain persisted, and once a week I went into the doctor's tiny office, located below ground in one of the oldest buildings on the medical school campus, to receive intravenous infusions and report any developments since my last visit.

I became a walking side effect: headaches from the infusions that were worse than the ones I took the drug to remedy, skin irritation wherever I applied the stuff, deepened exhaustion, dizziness that exacerbated the existing balance problems for which I already used a cane, nausea.

I'm still surprised that I survived. That Beverly survived.

§

Then I had the dream, after more than fifteen years of being sick: I dreamed that I was asleep dreaming that I was sick. Since I've been sick so long, I'm used to dreaming about being sick. The stalk of rotting celery, rooted deep within my body and growing out of my mouth. The slowing, stumbling walk that leads me into a vast crevasse through which I fall, twirling like an oak leaf and turning from green to red to gold as I near the bottom. The mirror in which I stare at my reflection without recognition. But now I was dreaming that I was dreaming that I was sick, a new turn in the labyrinth. Or rather, a new distancing, a dreamland effort that, at first, I understood to be saying *oh please, let it all have been a dream.* Since being sick so long is itself like a dream, this dream was a dream of a dream-reality twice removed. What's happened to me didn't really happen, or is only happening on another plane, or only to my body and not to me. It will vanish as soon as I wake up.

I really *thought* I had the whole dream/reality thing worked out. That I wasn't about to wake up and find it all had been just a nightmarish *Twilight Zone* episode. That I'd long ago accepted the facts of my illness and reconciled the obvious truth that my body and mind are connected. But then there was this dream, which seemed to suggest that some part of my mind still clung to the notion that this was all a chimera, the illness was something that would go away if perhaps I only changed my state of consciousness.

Was the dream some kind of cockamamie affirmation, showing that my true self was unaffected by the illness or by all the rippling fallout of treatments I'd tried? I already knew there were places inside me that none of this touched, that illness didn't reach. But that didn't mean my life-in-the-body was spared its actual pain, its compromised neurological operations, its many failures of function. There are multiple levels of reality at work in all this. The dream, I came to believe, was a metaphor for the selves I was trying to bring together, the one who was limited by his disabilities and the one— the master dreamer—who was imagining how to operate, how to slip out of the dream, despite the dreamland scenario in which he'd found himself. I was now well along the path of repossessing my body, even with its ongoing symptoms, rather than yielding it to the cascading rush of drugs and procedures.

I knew I wasn't going to be cured, I knew I was going to have to live with the aftermath of the viral attack, I knew I had to balance symptoms against the side effects of treatments for those symptoms, blah blah blah. It was all about side effects. Even my symptoms, I think, are essentially side effects of having survived the 1988 viral attack. I had to find the point where having control over symptoms tipped against losing control to side effects, and make choices. That, for me, became the imperative, the central treatment issue.

Without consciously choosing to, I'd been moving steadily away from traditional medical approaches and was using more alternative approaches. I underwent a five-day Ayurvedic detoxification program involving brisk rubdowns and enemas and herbalized steam inhalations and hot oil drips and music, all of which left me unchanged except that I needed to wear a diaper for a few days. I had—and still have—regular acupuncture, deep massage, homeopathic remedies, naturopathic remedies, chiropractic and osteopathic adjustments, all of which bring temporary relief. And minimal side effects.

In the dream's aftermath, convinced that the real side effect of all the side effects I'd endured was choosing to reclaim my body, I decided to learn ballroom dance. My dermatologist was getting married in late summer, her invitation had said there would be dancing, and I was going to try. Beverly and I bought two videos and I struggled to convert what I saw on the screen, where teachers would say, "Start with your right foot," but start with the foot that was to my left as I watched. Then I'd see our reflections in the living room window and be doubly confused. The rise and fall of a waltz made me lose balance, as did twirling in the western swing, but Beverly figured out that I'd remain stable as long as her hand remained in contact with me somewhere and my eyes remained locked on hers.

At the wedding reception, of course, the band played nothing but rock. This affirmed my deep post-illness belief that it was impossible to prepare for reality. We walked onto the dance floor, which was so crowded that even if I lost my balance I wouldn't fall. We put on the sunglasses that had been placed near every guest's plate so we would get into the spirit of Blues Brothers cool, or so we'd feel anonymous if we made fools of ourselves. And we danced, the only ones on the floor doing western swing to the rock music. It hurt and I stumbled, unable to see where my feet were going, but gradually the other dancers made room for us and I never let go of Beverly. Though I may have been in a world of my own, others were there with me and I knew I wasn't dreaming.

9

REVERTIGO

I can't find my hazelwood cane. It's not in the downstairs closet by our front door, where I was sure I'd stashed it two and a half years ago. It isn't in the car, where it had remained during all the months I needed it, nor in my office closet upstairs, the final resting place for stuff I can't part with. I bend and lean to reach behind a box of books by the closet wall, in case the cane has fallen back there. It hasn't, but now I have, hitting my head against the edge of a shelf, cutting the skin, raising an instant bump.

I fall because the world is awhirl. For the last three hours, since I woke up at 6:15, I've been overwhelmed by vertigo. Absolutely no warning signs. I got out of bed and the room was spinning. I lurched to the bathroom and back, grabbing at walls and doorframes for support against the swaying and swirling all around me. I had to kneel on the floor to put on my shirt, and I stumbled when I rose. I could barely make it downstairs for breakfast, holding onto the banister, concentrating on each step, and was too nauseous to eat anyway. All solid objects seemed like optical illusions, veering out of place as I approached or touched them. Trying to keep my head still, moving only my eyes, I could feel my back and shoulders tightening up, forming a shell.

At 8:30 I phoned my doctor's triage nurse, who found a 9:45 slot for me on the schedule. Now Beverly is ready to drive us there, but I can't find my cane and am not sure how far I can walk without falling. It's got to be here someplace. The cane had been too important to me for too long. I'd never get rid of it.

෨

From December 1988, when the viral attack targeted my brain, until the late spring of 2004, I couldn't walk without a cane. Through those fifteen years, the process of achieving balance and stability—slow as it was—progressed more steadily and seemed more likely to succeed than the process of managing my damaged memory systems or powers of cognition. Even now I'll sometimes stagger when I think, or hobble and blunder when I speak. So getting free of the cane had felt like a huge victory for me.

Once I'd weaned myself from it, for the next three and a half years I kept the cane in our car, just in case. Then one morning, as Beverly and I were loading our bikes into the cargo area for an autumn ride along the river, I'd noticed my cane's tip jutting from the cocoon of an old blanket tucked against the back seat. Yakking about the end of an era, feeling fully confident of my balance, I put the thing away at last, certain it was one of those moments I'd always remember. *The Storing of the Cane.*

Except when you have brain damage, you can't really be sure you'll remember anything, ever. I know that, deep in my being. It's why I have pens and pads in every room, in pockets, in the car. It's why I've trained myself, over the twenty-two years since I got sick, to write notes all the time, lists, reminders, things-to-do, ideas, phrases or images I don't want to lose. But I didn't write down where I put the hazelwood cane, since I was confident its location was emblazoned in my memory by the momentousness of the occasion. Besides, the cane was now a memento rather than a necessity. I could let it go.

Beverly and I had bought it together in Rapallo, Italy, during our honeymoon, to replace the stout oak cane I'd been using. With its long, thick, right-angled handle and slightly-too-long staff, its heaviness and density, the old cane had never felt comfortable. I'd picked it out before I understood what I really needed in a cane, and before I knew it would be with me for so long. When Beverly and I saw the pale, slender hazelwood cane propped in a shop window, we both smiled. Inside, we watched as the sweet old proprietor fit it perfectly to my five-foot-four frame, went into a back room to saw it down, and with an expression of deep sorrow, showed me the huge remnant he would be tossing away. This wasn't just an appliance, it was a thing of beauty, light and graceful and gnarled, the bark partially peeled, the handle ending in a knob that became polished over time by the oils of my hand.

🌀

Through those fifteen years when I needed the cane, my problem was a failure of my brain to assemble information about where I was in space, about what I saw or felt, about my body's relationship to whatever place it was in. I could see just fine; my skin and nerves and muscles all functioned well enough; the delicate bones and hair cells of my inner ear worked. But my brain couldn't properly sort what all these elements of the vestibular system were reporting. I'd fall sometimes when wind changed direction or when light flickered, when I reached the bottom—or occasionally the top—of a staircase, when landscape varied, patterns of floor coverings changed, or I was distracted by sound or movement. I might walk outside, savoring the spring air, and breathe in deeply, an action that sent me teetering backward. I'd squat to look at a freshly opened tulip, and fall into its embrace. Occasionally my world spun (vertigo) and occasionally my head spun (dizziness), the result of my brain being an inefficient machine for maintaining stability. I used to think Steve Martin could do a terrific routine about someone like me, deadly serious as he staggered and swooned and reeled through the world.

So I'm familiar with how it feels to live without balance, how vertigo floods the whole body. How being off-kilter alienates you from the world, even from its most familiar and reliable spaces such as your home. But this time, my vertigo is more pronounced, less mingled with other symptoms, and more relentless.

If vertigo came with a soundtrack, it would sometimes be train or trolley wheels grinding and screeching on tracks as the car turns and almost tips over. Other times it would be a treetop filled with the ruckus of rioting crows in a sudden windstorm. Helpless, untethered, I keep feeling the urge to reach out for something still and stable to steady me, but there's too much give in everything. I move through my carnival world like the Human Bumper Car while the core sensation recalls the belly's weightless hollow when a Ferris wheel plunges backward. If I weren't so out-of-balance, I think, I could walk the line between queasy and nauseous with more authority. Moving my head, changing its plane, sets everything in motion. Discord rules.

§

Not counting the two narrow closets in Beverly's art studio, where I would never store anything, there are six closets in our house. Time is running out before we have to leave, but I check each one. Since looking up or down makes me wobble, I do a lot of reaching into corners, onto shelves, back against walls, while holding my head steady. I feel like a poorly maintained robot.

The cane is not in my bedroom closet. It's not in the linen closet (surprise!) or guest room closet where Beverly's weaving materials are stored. It's not in the tiny, triangular hall closet whose packed shelves fill all available space. It's not in the pantry among the canned goods and vacuum cleaner and brooms and household tools. I check the downstairs closet by our front door again, because I'm still sure it's there even though I couldn't—and still can't—find it, despite examining every inch. Neither could Beverly, who has been going through the closets too.

On the way to our car, I inspect the garage systematically, all four corners, then along the walls, then up to the shelves that dangle from the ceiling, which makes me fall back against the door. Beverly takes my hand to steady me, and I see her eyes scan the space around the furnace, the recycling bins, the trash bucket.

Caneless, I go to my doctor and am told that I have benign paroxysmal positional vertigo, or BPPV, caused most likely by a coxsackie virus that has attacked my inner ear. He's seen four cases this week alone. He explains that ear rocks—small calcium carbonate crystals dislodged by the infection—have collected within my right inner ear. This debris, or otoconia, sends all sorts of confusing signals through the balance system, and until they dissolve I can expect the imbalance, vertigo, light-headedness, and nausea to continue. To last anywhere, he says, putting a hand on my shoulder, from two days to two months and, perhaps, to recur in the future.

First thing I do when I get home is check all six closets again. Then I check them yet again. I do it slowly each time, fighting both vertigo and a growing sense of disbelief. I know the cane is here somewhere. It doesn't make sense, and I'm going to keep looking until I find it. Because I'm tired of things in my environment not making sense already. *'Tis all in pieces, all coherence gone,* as Donne wrote in "An Anatomy of the World." Reason, logic, systematic investigation, that's what's called for. A little coherence, please. I sense that I'm enacting a kind of behavioral vertigo with this reeling, zany pursuit, but can't stop myself.

I move the same coats, shoes, boxes, bathrobes, bedding, yarns, pillows, brooms, tools, cans, mailing tubes, fans, appliances, that I moved before. I feel along the same walls and same suspicious corners. There it is! No, that's the umbrella I've mistaken for the cane three times now.

On the second search, I work in the opposite direction, starting upstairs instead of downstairs, going through each closet from the right instead of the left, as though these shenanigans will make a difference in the outcome. Magical thinking. Which seems called for, since regular thinking isn't getting the results I need. While I'm upstairs, Beverly is downstairs, re-rechecking closet and pantry, reporting her nonfindings.

I forage through the garage again, frisking the wicker shelves where we store, folded over itself, the flowery-patterned cushion for our outdoor chaise longue; boxes of Christmas ornaments from Beverly's childhood; boxes of candles; and recycled orange juice containers for Beverly's basket-making dyes. I have no idea why I think the cane would be hidden in the bag where we keep our inflatable kayak, but I check anyway. No luck. The cane is also still not hidden behind the stepladder. Not behind the bicycles or the coat rack crowded with winter wear or the luggage, so it hasn't relocated itself when I wasn't looking.

Since I can do nothing about the vertigo, since even lying down quietly doesn't make it go away—in fact, makes it worse once I get up again—and since the simple and familiar order of a stable world is missing, I know I'm searching for something more than just a vanished cane here. I'm after control, after normalcy, clarity, an end to this dreamworld scenario. But I am also after the cane, and for a while I can keep justifying my mad, vertiginous, ongoing quest.

After yet another fruitless round through the six closets, and after a desperate investigation of Beverly's two sacrosanct art studio closets, I get into bed and settle back against a stack of five pillows to keep my head elevated. I read my *Merck Manual*'s understated, dull, utterly inadequate definition of vertigo: "an abnormal sensation of rotary movement associated with difficulty in balance, gait, and navigation of the environment." But then it talks about "the hallucination of movement of the environment," a notion accurately suggesting the sort of trippy, altered-state feeling I can't shake. I read my *Encyclopedia of Medicine*: "astronauts in zero gravity experience vertigo when moving their heads." Yes, zero gravity, that's also what this feels like. Adrift in space. I reread a little of Scott McCredie's *Balance: In Search of the Lost Sense*. He says that we depend on our balance system "not only for maintaining an upright posture, but for vision and even mental acuity," which explains, perhaps, why I've been behaving so stupidly. When things are so wildly out of balance outside our heads, I think, things quickly get out of balance inside our heads too. I feel—after just one morning of this—as though I'm not myself. It's a feeling I find echoed in Oliver Sacks's *The Man Who Mistook His Wife for a Hat*, where he writes about a woman who lost the power of proprioception, the sense of her body's whereabouts in space: "There is this specific, organically based, feeling of disembodiedness." I'm disembodied, but also trapped in my body.

None of this is particularly comforting. So I get up and start checking closets again.

೫

Beverly and I are doing *The Epley Maneuver*. Named after Oregon ear surgeon John Epley, who invented the technique nearly thirty years ago, it involves a series of four precise head movements intended to relocate the inner ear debris that causes symptoms in people with BPPV. *The Particle Repositioning Procedure*. We read about it online, watched a couple of YouTube demonstrations, and called my doctor to ask if he thought it would help. He did. Or, to be more precise about his phrasing, he thought it might not hurt.

Now I'm lying back on our bed, head turned to the right and dangling off the edge into Beverly's hands. This makes me even dizzier, but the feeling passes as Beverly waits thirty seconds, then shifts my head to the left. After another thirty seconds, I rotate onto my left side, face down, and look at Beverly's kneecap. When another thirty seconds pass, I slowly sit up and gather myself for a full minute, trying not to puke. Repeat three times a day.

At least we're doing something! I've already implemented *The Don't Sleep on the Right Side Program*. Now we follow *The Epley Maneuver* with *The Ginger Tea Operation*, to calm my stomach. Then Beverly gets out her acupuncture needles. She'd studied the practice for a year, during the time she was a licensed massage therapist, and we're both confident that her treatments can help ease my symptoms.

After all this, I feel sure I'll be able to find my cane. Because while I was lying in bed with needles in my hands, arms, legs, and the top of my head, I had a vision: the cane was in plain sight, blending with its surroundings like a cuttlefish. It was camouflaged; that's why I couldn't find it.

I check beside, behind, and underneath every piece of wooden furniture. In the space between the wall and the six-shelf bookcase in our bedroom, I find my old wooden baseball bat, the one I kept beside our bed for security when we lived in the woods for thirteen years. Too heavy, short, and awkwardly shaped for a cane. Under the futon in our guest bedroom, I find a few tangles of thin reed Beverly uses to make baskets. In the two-inch gap between my desk and wall,

I find a missing coaster and a small ruler. The almost-cane-shaped thing behind the family room credenza is still our fireplace poker, still made of metal, still black, still not my cane.

I'm beginning to understand what Samuel Beckett meant when he wrote of a man who *spangled the butterflies of vertigo*. I'm flitting; the world sparkles me dizzy as nothing holds still, and the vertigo increases as I whirl around in pursuit of stability. I also grasp what Charles Baudelaire said in early 1862, after suffering continually from vertigo: "I have felt the wind of the wing of madness pass over me." It's not just that vertigo's symptoms are driving me crazy, they reveal the madness of a world that no longer makes sense. All is illusion. What is stillness but another illusion, since Earth is always in motion? This feeling that all is illusion, that stillness is really just another form of motion, must be why Milan Kundera said, in *The Unbearable Lightness of Being*, that vertigo "is the voice of the emptiness below us."

It's nearing noon. Time for the next *Epley Maneuver*. Beverly positions the pillow and clock, kneels, and tells me to lean back. Cupping my head in her hands, she looks down and asks how I'm doing. I feel the breath of her voice over my face. That's when I start to cry.

I feel engulfed by gratitude for her love and tenderness, for the great good fortune of not being alone as I deal with this. But also, having felt both physical and behavioral vertigo, I'm now feeling emotional vertigo. I'm swamped. This is good, I know it is, but crying just makes my head feel more clogged and imbalanced.

When I sit up, Beverly gives me a tissue and I blow my nose. The shift in sinus pressure doesn't make my vertigo vanish, but it does give me a sudden insight: I've been approaching the search for my cane, and thus for support, for stability, all wrong. Too much action—all the leaning and crouching and reaching keeps making me fall, which should have been a sign that I needed to find another way—and not enough looking.

After lunch, I head to the garage. No matter how many times I think about it, this is the last place I can actually remember having the cane in my hands. I turn on the fluorescent lights, stand beside the car, and stare. My eye is caught by how much the patterned cushion folded up on our wicker shelving looks like camouflage, and that's when I see the rounded tip of the cane's cream-colored knob protruding from within the fold. It appears to be little more than a detail of the cushion's flower shapes, barely a shade lighter than its surrounding fabric.

My first thought is that there's no way my cane could fit on that shelf. Am I really *that* short? It turns out that the cane measures thirty-two and a half inches from tip to knob, and the shelf measures thirty-two inches from its left rear corner to its right front edge. My cane was 98 percent swallowed up by the folded cushion. It turns out that I *am* that short.

Like King Arthur with Excalibur, I withdraw the cane from its hold and heft it once. Though I'm not suddenly imbued with magical powers, and though the vertigo doesn't vanish, I'm impressed with how familiar and comfortable it feels to have the cane's support. Also with how confident it makes me feel, at last, that I'll get through this, as though the cane were the missing piece of the arsenal, along with *The Epley Maneuver* and Beverly's support and ginger tea and acupuncture and patience and time.

Metaphors swarm. Though I may feel overwhelmed, swallowed up by vertigo like my cane was swallowed by the cushion, there's a crucial piece of me where stability remains intact and available. The quiet center. And I know how to find it, how to lead myself there, where balance and harmony are to be found, even if I'm not aware that I'm doing so: I write, or if I can't write I make notes, even if the notes are little more than single words or phrases, trying to understand what's happening to me; I turn to Beverly; I phone my daughter. I gather what I need to keep myself together.

The truth is, since the still world is always spinning, always in motion, our bodies and brains and minds work together to sustain the illusion of stability, to hold ourselves steady without thinking about it. That's our system of balance at work, attuned, flexible, silent, in the background. But our hold is tenuous, and not guaranteed. In this sense, I've come to see my encounters with vertigo and dizziness, with illnesses that strike at the core of my balance, as a peek beyond the familiar dimensions of my grip on earth. Or perhaps behind the curtain, or through the magician's cloak, since all that holds us in place is really just a trick of eye, ear, skin, muscle, and bone.

The cane doesn't fix me, but it helps hold me in place. Being able to walk more confidently enables me to feel less helpless and to avoid additional fall-related injury. After a month, though the symptoms persist and I'm still reeling, I imagine celebrating someday as I put my cane back in a place I will never forget. I try to remain hopeful. We continue doing *The Epley Maneuver* three times a day.

It takes another month to realize that, since *The Epley Maneuver* isn't resolving the problem, the problem might not be caused by BPPV.

10

SWAY ME SMOOTH

Soundtrack for an MRI of the Brain

I Like to Move It

"Don't move," the technician named Molly says. Then she squeezes
my ankle and leaves the room. Move? I'm supine, with a thick white
semicircular cage locked across my entire face. Rubber chocks im-
mobilize my neck and head on a table so narrow I think one deep
breath could topple me. Even if I weren't still dizzy. But I've been
dizzy nonstop now for thirteen weeks and six days. When I lie, sit,
stand. When I look up or down, left or right. When wind stirs the
maple leaves outside my bedroom window or birds fly by or images
flash on the television screen. I can't drive, still need a cane, have fallen
in grocery stores and on sidewalks. And now I'm in a remodeled
former cake factory, about to be drawn into the bore of a giant
magnet. The magnet will force the hydrogen atoms in my brain to
line up neatly, then bombard them with radio waves so a computer

can identify what's causing the problem in my brain or inner ear. Movement is something I'm no longer good at, and no longer do without careful planning. So okay, Molly, I won't move.

Suddenly her voice is in my head. "Earphones work?"

I force myself not to nod, and risk a shallow-breathed whisper. "Unless I'm having aural hallucinations."

"Good. Now what kind of music do you like?"

Like most people, my head is often filled with music. Broadway, 1950s rock, the pop crooners, dance music. A random word can trigger a whole string of melody and lyrics, which explains why the song running through my brain now, triggered a moment ago by Molly saying "don't move," is once again Reel 2 Real's 1994 hit "I Like to Move It." It was a sticky song—an earworm—for me even before Beverly and I watched Julianne Hough and Apolo Anton Ono samba to it on *Dancing with the Stars*. *I like to move it, move it. I like to move it, move it.*

"Music?"

"Yeah, we can play music through your earphones. Helps distract you. Some of the scans can be a little noisy."

A little noisy. I've had two brain MRIs before, twenty years ago, and remember feeling like I was stuck inside a jackhammer.

Without thinking, and overriding the crazed tune in my head, I tell Molly "the old standards." That seems to confound her. There's a click in my earphones, then silence, then another click.

"Name a singer you like."

I didn't think she'd know who Vaughn Monroe was. Or Matt Monro either. "Well, how about Michael Bublé?"

"That'll work."

She reminds me about the squeeze ball she handed me to use if I need help, and re-reminds me not to move. Then the table is sliding backward and I know enough to close my eyes so I won't have to see the tiny space where I'll be spending the next forty-five minutes.

Molly's view of me now: the pale blue paper shorts I've been issued, from which protrude my legs and feet held absolutely still.

Feeling Good

Google the phrase "MRI noise" and you find a range of descriptions: banging, beeping, buzzing, clanging, clicking, grinding, hammering, knocking, tapping, whirring. But the adjective preceding those descriptions is consistent: loud. And, for brain images, that loud noise is scant inches from your ears.

According to howstuffworks.com, an MRI's noise is caused by "the rising electrical current in the wires of the gradient magnets being opposed by the main magnetic field. The stronger the main field, the louder the gradient noise." Or, as the Boston *Globe* explains, "the fact that the strength of the magnet has to be changed over time and position means that all sorts of things move at least a bit in response to it, and that motion makes sound—that clanging noise." As it scans to generate several sets of images, the MRI's noise changes volume and intensity, producing a variety of decibel levels.

The Lancet, among the world's leading independent general medical journals, says an MRI peaks at between 122 and 131 decibels. That's just a little bit louder than a nearby thunderclap (120), or about the level of a jet at takeoff (130). Sometimes during a procedure the decibel level is between 90 and 100, or like lying beside a lawnmower (85–90), motorcycle (88), or farm tractor (98). As the National Institute on Deafness and Other Communication Disorders notes, "Regular exposure to sound over 100 dB of more than one minute risks permanent hearing loss."

But I'm wearing earphones and, for distraction from the racket, will be listening to tunes. I've removed my gold and hematite earring so the magnets won't rip my ear off. I have no pacemaker or artificial joints, so the procedure shouldn't suck my heart or shoulder out of my body. Everything's under control. As I settle into the machine's isocenter and reposition the squeeze ball against my belly, the first scan begins. I'd call this one a snowmobile (105).

After a minute or two passes—*did she forget the music?*—and very faintly within the riot of sound surrounding me, I can hear music (decibel level of rustling leaves: 20, the threshold for "just audible"). That's it? All I get is rustling leaves? *A little volume in here, Moll.* Is this worth squeezing the ball about? Then slowly, the volume comes up and there's Michael Bublé singing that great old Broadway number "Feeling Good."

Well, I *had* been feeling good, particularly for a man of sixty-one disabled since 1988 by a virus that had targeted his brain. I'd had a stable, healthy winter and first days of spring. Faulty balance was one aftermath of the viral attack that I no longer worried about. The way I'd been looking at it, I would never reclaim losses to my cognitive powers, memory, or abstract reasoning capacity, would never have a reliable immune system, but I'd learned how to live with what remained, and I was steady on my feet. *It's a new life / for me.*

Till that early spring morning in 2009. *Blossom on a tree / You know how I feel.* I'd spent a weekend at the Oregon coast, where I'd caught a cold, but I was starting to feel better, was *driftin' on by.* But then I folded back the sheets on the morning of March 27, got out of bed, and found the world whirling counterclockwise. It also felt as though I'd been pushed or tripped by a ghost lurking beside the bed. But even when I was on all fours, the vertigo didn't stop. I made it back into bed and, showing keen analytical insight, told Beverly "something's wrong."

In about three hours, we were at my internist's office. After diagnosing BPPV, he said, "We don't really know what triggers it. Might be viral, might be weather related, might be age, trauma. Did you hit your head?"

"Not that I remember."

He laughed, then shrugged and said, "I see a lot of BPPV in the spring."

It was a reasonable diagnosis, certainly the most likely explanation for my symptoms and their sudden onset. BPPV is the most common cause of vertigo. But as the projected two-month duration was ending, and none of the remedies we tried were working, I finally admitted what I'd been thinking about: the diagnosis was likely to have been incorrect. After all, my vertigo wasn't paroxysmal, since it didn't come and go, but remained constant no matter what I did. Or didn't do. Sometimes I might be awhirl, sometimes everything around me was awhirl, and sometimes nothing whirled but I was so light-headed that I seemed to be floating away. So if it wasn't paroxysmal, and it didn't have anything to do with position, and it wasn't only vertigo, and it no longer felt benign, maybe it wasn't benign paroxysmal positional vertigo after all. My doctor agreed it was time to see a balance specialist.

And this old world is a new world. That's right, focus on the music. Thinking about the diagnostic journey is making me restless. "Feeling Good" is a song I remember from the Broadway show *The Roar of the Greasepaint—The Smell of the Crowd*, which I saw when I was eighteen. It was all about getting the Man to Share the Power, Freedom for the Worker. Very sixties. Who was in that? British guy, actor/singer, was on all the talk shows. Married to what's-her-name. Wait, wait, Joan Collins. Anthony Newley! I'm pleased to nail the actor's name, under the circumstances, and then I get a bonus: I remember that he cowrote the songs. Even if Newley gave us the saccharine "Candy Man" and "Talk to the Animals," and all the angst of "Who Can I Turn To?" and "What Kind of Fool Am I?" he did manage to write "Feeling Good." Reedy-voiced, charming, emotional Anthony Newley. Music is performing its magic on me here, triggering memories and releasing feelings. I'm getting relaxed, *feeling good*—great idea to have this piped in music—but I'm also having trouble keeping still as Michael Bublé gets the song swinging toward its conclusion. *Oh freedom is mine!* How weird to hear a celebration of freedom while transfixed and caged inside a horizontal tube. What I want at this instant, almost irresistibly, is to snap my fingers or shake my jazz hands. According to Oliver Sacks in his 2007 book *Musicophilia*, "Listening to music is not just auditory and emotional, it is motoric as well. 'We listen to music with our muscles,' as Nietzsche wrote. We keep time to music, involuntarily." So of course I can't help needing to move. Dance music in an MRI. I wonder if just wiggling my toes a little will violate Molly's command.

Sway

The MRI machine is named Tim, after its Total Imaging Matrix technology. This, according to the manufacturer, Siemens, provides "advanced image detail and speed, scanning flexibility, and power." But Tim is a real loudmouth, so I can't at first identify the new song that's playing.

Oh, it's "Sway," Pablo Beltrán Ruiz's great mambo from 1953. I've loved this song and known Norman Gimbel's English lyrics since I was a kid with dreams of being a crooner. But hold on, this isn't Michael Bublé's version. *Pipe down, Tim.* The combination of being dizzy, being inundated with CLANGING HAMMERING I THINK WE'RE AT THE POWER-SAW LEVEL (110) noise, trying to concentrate on identifying the singer while not responding to the music, and feeling confused, makes me suddenly queasy. If the nausea gets any worse, I may have to squeeze the ball and get out of here.

It's Dino! I recognize the soused-sounding baritone of Dean Martin and remember trying to imitate it as a thirteen-year-old boy. I'd wanted to learn the sexy song's lyrics so I could add it to my repertoire for when my voice finished changing. *Molly, this is a mambo, for God's sake, and you want me not to move. What are you doing to me?*

I try to settle down but, as the current scan intensifies, the table starts vibrating. *Tim, you're not on the beat here.* Surely this happens all the time, isn't a sign of impending catastrophe, and doesn't count against the Don't Move commandment. *Like a lazy ocean hugs the shore / Hold me close, sway me more.* I feel trapped between the urge to move with the song's rhythm and resistance to random movement from the table's vibration.

But it's better than being in the Omniax System chair, where in early June I was spun upside down and sideways by the famous neurotologist, who then diagnosed me with endolymphatic hydrops instead of BPPV. It had taken me two weeks to get an appointment at his balance clinic, and I had to pay for all costs myself because he wouldn't accept Medicare patients, but I'd looked forward to gaining clarity about what was wrong with me.

The Omniax looks like a futuristic (and expensive) carnival ride, or a device for training astronauts to endure zero-gravity. Inside an open, circular metal frame, there's a high-backed seat festooned with straps. Harnessed like a fighter pilot in a cockpit, wearing a goggle-tipped headset equipped with infrared cameras, I was swiveled, twirled, somersaulted, and backflipped through full circles across several planes. I was also shifted sideways and suddenly upright, dangled, rotated. Through those maneuvers, the cameras revealed that I had none of benign paroxysmal positional vertigo's characteristic nystagmus, the jerky involuntary eye movements caused when ear rocks get shaken up by movement of the head. Therefore I had a definitive un-diagnosis: not BPPV. And was now dizzier than I imagined possible. *When we sway I go weak.*

What followed were two days of tests spaced a week apart. I stood on floors that were suddenly tilted or jerked in different directions, and challenged to maintain equilibrium. My eyes and ears were tested with flashing lights and weird head movements, with blowing air and pure tones. Electrodes were stuck deep into my ears to record brain stem response to sounds, and onto my forehead and neck to test the inner ear's response to clicks and short bursts of sound when I turned my head.

According to his report, the neurotologist found my acoustic reflexes "suggestive of diffuse cochlear disease." My eyes didn't work—separately or together—as head position changed: "The patient drops visual acuity five lines when moving his head to the left and three lines when moving his head to the right (both abnormal)." I showed "a marked vestibular deficit type of postural dyscontrol with somatosensory dependence" and my ability to adapt to movement underfoot was "impaired." In other words, technology and medical science confirmed that I WAS DIZZY. My balance system was measurably a mess, and I wasn't making it up.

To the expert, it was a result of endolymphatic hydrops, a vestibular disorder caused by abnormal fluctuations in the fluid of the inner ear. Those fluids, normally maintained at constant volume and chemical consistency, keep the sensory cells that control balance functioning properly. Something had caused the volume and composition of my fluids to change.

"By far the most likely cause of his hydrops," he wrote, "is a viral endolabyrinthitis." He thought that either a reactivation of the virus that had damaged my brain twenty years earlier or a reactivation of the chicken pox virus I'd caught in 2002 were the likeliest culprits.

With a prescription for powerful antiviral drugs, a book about dietary management of hydrops, and a plan for months of vestibular rehabilitation in hand, I went home and called my internist for a follow-up appointment. I was not about to take Valtrex without his approval. And besides, what did he think of this diagnosis and treatment plan?

He smiled as soon as I uttered the first two syllables of endolymphatic, so I stopped talking, handed him the prescription, and tried not to move my head as he talked. It wasn't surprising that a specialist who sees so many patients with one particular disease would diagnose me as having that disease. My internist had done the same thing with me earlier, finding a different and even more common balance disorder. But I didn't have the full range of symptoms for endolymphatic hydrops: no sense of pressure or fullness in the ears, no ringing or roaring sounds, no hearing loss. And my dizziness and vertigo didn't vary the way they would if my problem were based on inner ear fluid fluctuations. They were always present.

So he called his friend, a neurologist who specializes in balance problems. I could get in to see him four days later, June 30. At our first meeting, he watched me approach, my head held rigidly, my shoulders hunched, my hand gripping the cane, and nodded. "You look like a dizzy man."

It's happening again. Thinking about how hard it's been to find out what's wrong with me, and why, is making me more agitated. But what's a person to think about during an MRI that might finally reveal the truth. Even if it's a truth I'm not eager to know, such as a tumor or stroke in the brain stem, as the neurologist casually mentioned. "Let's have a look," he said, patting me on the shoulder, "so we can rule things out."

Sing to me, Dino. I need you now. He might be able to *hear the sounds of violins* but right now I'm hearing sounds that remind me of the subways of my Brooklyn childhood (88 dB). The train of doom.

I realize I'm much more comfortable fighting the immediate battle against mambo-inspired movement than thinking about the diagnostic herky-jerk I've been doing since March 27. Come on, Dino, *sway me smooth, sway me now.*

They Can't Take That Away from Me

About a half hour through the MRI, I make a mistake. As the silence after the end of Tony Bennett's "I Left My Heart in San Francisco" extends, and another scan (mild, maybe only an 80- decibel garbage disposal) winds down, Molly clicks back on and says, "How you doing in there?" I react to her sudden presence by opening my eyes, something I didn't want to do.

The immediate view is of a small rectangular mirror mounted inside the cage over my face. It can't be more than two or three inches away, and is angled so I can see into that part of the room framed by the tube's opening but nearly blocked by my toes. There's nothing to see but a glimpse of white wall. I know that Molly and another technician are in a room there, watching me through a window just above my view. Peripheral vision lets me see that the sides of the tube are even closer than I imagined. I shut my eyes.

"I'm okay."

"One more scan, then we'll pull you out and inject dye for the last images. Hang on."

The procedure has seemed to go on for hours, yet I'm surprised to hear that it's almost over already. Time has both stood still and flown by. Past and present have folded together too. It's as though the rearranging of magnetic fields in here has shattered the familiar bounds of time. Which is another way of saying that there's so much we don't know about the workings of the human brain. Not just the experience of time, but also—and obviously—the experience of space, the intricacies of identifying where the body is and how it maintains equilibrium. Neurology knows the basics, and the way much of the wiring operates, but there are substantial mysteries remaining, especially when the system malfunctions and the customary explanations fail.

The next scan begins with a few gentle clanks and pings, as though Tim is clearing his throat. I tune him out. Immersed in the mix of music and noise, with my eyes shut, I've been turned deeply inward during much of the MRI, dwelling in the past rather than the present, following the flow of memory. The songs I heard triggered associations, shifted mood, loosened imagination. They took me away from here. And for a while they counteracted the great feelings of loss, dislocation, and disorientation that accompany both long-term illness and the kind of sudden, life-changing episode embodied by my vertigo. Despite the discomfort and annoyance of the MRI procedure, I was having a pretty good time here.

These thoughts, as one of my favorite Gershwin songs starts playing within a ruckus rising to maybe the 75-decibel level of a dishwasher next to my ears, feel revelatory. They remind me of how much I retain despite the things that are wrong with me, how sustained I am by music, by Beverly and the love we share, by friendship. *No, no—they can't take that away from me.*

From the moment I lost my balance, Beverly has been a kind of spirit level showing me the way to find steadiness despite what was happening inside my brain. As Frank Sinatra sings *the way your smile just beams* I remember looking up at Beverly's smile so many times during our futile repetitions of *The Epley Maneuver.* From my position, though her smile was shaped like a frown, I saw such tenderness that it made me cry. Which made her worry that I was losing hope. Just the opposite. *The way you've changed my life!*

A month ago, my friend George Core, after learning of my symptoms, sent me an Irish walking stick he'd had in his home in

Tennessee, a genuine shillelagh made of blackthorn and hazelwood. It arrived unexpectedly, just after lunch, packed in a long, thin box, and delivered to my door by Federal Express with a brief, warm note of support. My friend Hilda Raz encouraged me to go ahead and fly to Memphis for a long-planned visit with my daughter, saying that flying hadn't worsened her own symptoms of vertigo, which I didn't know she'd had. Within an hour of posting a note on Facebook about my condition, I received dozens of responses from people who'd either had the same thing or knew someone who did. I was buoyed by the sense that my situation, which had struck me as so bizarre and rare, turned out to be far more common than I supposed. I'd read the statistics, but until people in my life began to talk about their symptoms, I hadn't internalized the knowledge that vertigo strikes so many. Friends advised me, reassured me *on that bumpy road*, and now it felt like they were here with me again. Maybe that's why I felt so crammed in here.

Fever

Bublé's voice again, and the first lyrics I can distinguish, after the plucked bass and cymbal taps, are *never know how much I care*. Thank you, Michael. "Fever" transports me back to adolescence, when Peggy Lee's 1958 version of the song opened a whole new idea for me of what sex might be about. There was more than mechanics involved! And girls enjoyed it too! Then a couple years later, Elvis sang the song in a suave, knowing way that suggested it was possible—effective, even—to smolder quietly. This was a song to study, not just memorize.

But now it stops—just before we get to Romeo and Juliet, and the only occurrence of the word *forsooth* in popular music that I know of—and I'm being drawn out of the MRI. I hadn't realized how warm I felt until leaving the machine's confines for the cool air of the larger room. Molly, seeing gooseflesh, offers me a blanket.

As she begins preparing a vein in my arm for the contrast dye injection, I look away, toward the door beyond which Beverly waits. It refuses to hold steady, and I can feel myself being swept up in the kind of swooning spiral that's become a frequent sensation over these months. I think of it as an inner cyclone, and wonder if that's what L. Frank Baum had in mind when he began *The Wizard of Oz* with a cyclone that sweeps Dorothy out of the Kansas prairies and into a strange and alien land. Maybe Baum had vertigo. So what I need is a pair of Silver Shoes like Dorothy's. Then all I have to do is put them on, knock their heels together three times, and command them to return me to the place of balance. What, I wonder as Molly squeezes my ankle again and sends me back into the tube, would be the right song for that journey?

At Last

If I didn't know better, I'd say that Molly had this planned. As the final scan revs up like an outboard engine, the song that comes on is Etta James's version of "At Last." She's one of those blues singers, and "At Last" is one of those complexly romantic songs that I don't remember knowing about until I was in my forties, when I was ready for them.

Though I'm grateful that *at last, my love has come along*, and I know how fortunate I am, in this moment I take the song to suggest something else entirely. Not just that at last the MRI will be over. Not even that at last I may learn what's causing my symptoms, and find effective treatment. I'm thinking that all the signs are aligned—like the MRI has aligned my hydrogen molecules, like the playlist is ending with a song called "At Last" that's about bad fortune coming to an end—to reveal a hidden truth: I will get better. That's the *dream that I can call my own.*

Now that this occurs to me, I see a trend starting a week ago. Things fell into place as they almost never do: I called my internist at just the right time for him to call the neurologist so the neurologist could see me for his last available appointment before his annual month-long vacation. Having heard the report from my internist and given me a quick exam, he set up this MRI, requested test results from the neurotologist, and would call me with results before leaving town. He even had the same name as my best friend from childhood in Brooklyn.

Easy, I tell myself as the MRI ends; maybe I'm reaching for meaning where there's only coincidence. Side effect of having my brain zapped by magnets. But I get off the table feeling optimistic. *Feeling good.*

Over the Rainbow

The neurologist calls to say my MRI reveals no sign of stroke or tumor. Looks to him like there's a slight area of contact between a blood vessel and nerves of the inner ear. Maybe that's the cause. I'm in no danger—unless I fall, so I should be careful—and he'll see me after he returns from vacation. He also says I should take a tiny dose, just a half milligram, of Valium twice a day to dampen the nerve responses. See you August 24.

Through July and early August, I take my Valium and notice no significant change in symptoms. At the grocery store, I bend to reach a roll of paper towels, stand, turn toward my cart, lose my balance, and fall sideways. The shillelagh clatters to the floor, the package of paper towels goes flying behind me, and I'm so humiliated I want to bawl. Beverly helps me up. At the gas station, I start getting out of the car to clean the windshield and something—maybe a change of light in the air as clouds pass, maybe an unevenness in the concrete— makes me swoon backward into the car again.

At about eight on the evening of August 12, Beverly and I are sitting on the couch in our living room. It's been raining all day, unusual for Portland in the summer. I'm reading Willie Morris's memoir of his friendship with James Jones when suddenly there's a great burst of outward pressure inside my head. It plugs my ears and the world goes silent. I drop the book, open my mouth wide, put both hands to my ears. In two seconds, the pressure reverses, vanishes. My responses have caught Beverly's attention.

"Did something happen?"

I explain and, delighted that I can talk, that I can move both arms, can shift position on the couch, add, "I don't think it was a stroke."

She looks at me for several seconds, then smiles. "Stand up. I wonder if your dizziness is gone."

I do. It is. *And the dreams that you dare to dream / Really do come true.*

Twelve days later, the neurologist doesn't notice that I've walked into his consulting room without a cane. He doesn't notice that my shoulders and neck are no longer hunched down like someone afraid to move. When I tell him what happened, and that except for some residual light-headedness the symptoms haven't returned, he nods, then shakes his head.

"I'd like to take credit for this," he tells me, chuckling, "but I don't think I can." He's quiet for a few moments, then says, with a tone of amazement in his voice, "Those test results, and my own exam, I have to say you were in measurably poor vestibular shape." He's quiet again, looking out the window. "Based on what you just told me, I have a theory about what caused your symptoms."

For a moment, I'm actually not sure I want to hear this. Not that I believe in miracles there in the land of Oz where I'd dwelt for five months. But with all the diagnoses that turned out to be incorrect, and with all my ongoing admiration for the mysteries of neurological function, I'm not convinced I'll believe him. Then where will I be?

No, I have to hear this. I put my notebook on the desk and take out my pen, and look at him.

"Intracranial hypertension. On a molecular level, viruses are much larger than normal spinal fluid. Given your history, I'd say it's possible that an earlier virus reactivated, or you caught a new one, which caused a buildup of viral material in the spinal fluid, which plugged up the holes through which the fluid normally drains." He looks and sounds like he's testing the idea rather than confirming it. "Plugged drains led to a buildup of fluid and pressure, which caused the symptoms." His gaze returned to me. "I actually thought about this possibility before, and wondered what would happen if I gave you a spinal tap. Probably would have released the pressure and you'd have been fine."

"So it came unplugged on its own, twelve days ago?"

"It's a pretty elegant theory." He smiled again. "Listen, if your symptoms ever return, we'll do the tap right away and I bet it fixes you right up."

The symptoms still haven't returned. I look back to that rainy August night when the barometric pressure had changed so radically. I remember that earlier in the day I'd had another of the weekly acupuncture treatments I'd been taking for my dizziness. Weather? Needles? Spontaneous unplugging of viral material? They all sound both absurd and plausible—as did ear rocks and fluctuating fluids—as explanations for the distortion of my body's fragile system of balance that came and went so suddenly. What I know is that one night, as suddenly as I arrived there, I returned from the land of Oz without even having to click the heels of my Silver Shoes.

11

ANNIVERSARY FEVER

Day by nomadic day
Our anniversaries go by,
Dates anchored in an inner sky,
To utmost ground, interior clay.

Douglas Dunn,
from "Anniversaries"

Today's my father's birthday. He'd be 102. In four years, he'll have been dead as long as he was alive.

Today's also ten days before the first anniversary of the day I woke up, got out of bed, went reeling against the wall, and fell on my face. The vertigo lasted 138 days. It may have been brought on by reactivation of a virus that had targeted my brain 21 years earlier.

I never have recovered what I lost in cognitive function 21 years ago. Particularly in the realms of abstract reasoning, capacity to structure thought or visual stimuli, reliable word-finding ability, concentration, and memory. Last week, I announced to Beverly that I'd *numbed* the television rather than *muted* it. I also told her that I would *evaporate* rather than *delete* a film we'd just watched on our DVR. Last night, by the time I reached pen and notepad, I could no longer remember the item I'd wanted to add to our shopping list. This morning, because of their abstract nature, I couldn't even begin formulating answers to an interviewer's string of questions: *How have you thought about your-self in relation to writing? What are your thoughts about being an artist in 2010 in the United States, and how do you see the role of the artist?* Common enough occasional glitches for most people, especially as they age, but for me they have been typical of how I've functioned across the last 21 years.

Today's also eleven days before my maternal grandfather's birthday. He'd be 124. He was 94 when he died on Leap Day, February 29, 1980. Since the anniversary of his death date only comes around every 4 years, I keep trying to figure out how to compute the year in which he'll have been dead as long as he lived. Adding 94 years to his 1980 death would be 2074. But there's only one February 29 per 4 years, so . . . Can't do it. Too abstract, or too neuro-convoluted for me, for my damaged brain. Still, I try to work on puzzles like this, or like Sudoku, to stimulate my brain. Recent research has shown that our brains are more plastic than previously supposed, and that damaged brain cells can repair or regenerate themselves. So let's see, if it takes 4 years to accumulate 1 year on my grandfather's death-tally, and he died in 1980 at 94, would it take 376 years (4 x 94) for him to be dead for 94 years? So he'd be dead as long as he was alive in 2356? At which point I would be 409, or 221 years older than my grandfather.

While hoping to grow new brain cells, I also use, as a kind of mind-cane, various aids to compensate for and manage my cognitive losses. Scribblings on index cards, scraps of paper, and Post-it notes that I collect in multicolored folders to organize fragments of memory, thought, experience. Techniques of repetition and sensual association to help shift important memories from short-term to long-term storage: *Her name is Susan, his name is Herman, so Her-man is her man.* Rigorous control of distraction to enhance concentration: *No background music when reading or writing, no views of trees or birds from my desk.* Or an obsession with calendars and anniversaries to find and anchor myself in time, manage my broken sense of coherence, create a feeling of order. I know I go overboard with it, have a case of chronic anniversary fever. But for me, in a very urgent way, the philosophical idea that tormented T. S. Eliot in his poem "Burnt Norton" is a firm daily reality: "Time present and time past / Are both perhaps present in time future / And time future contained in time past." Time truly swirls through me. And memory, as Richard Lattimore described it in his poem "Anniversary," is but the "shell of moon / on day-sky, two o'clock in lazy June." I feel compelled— driven—to grab whatever I can, however faint, and hold it in mind.

When I can access a memory, revisit a person or experience, it's a kind of anniversary. The echoing moment, past but present, alive. It's the flip-side of what happens when an anniversary triggers the memory of a person or experience. The British poet Ted Hughes, recalling his mother's death in "Anniversary," writes that "Every May Thirteenth / I see her with her sister Miriam." In that poem, the recollection is stimulated by Hughes quite purposefully: "I lift / The torn-off diary page where my brother jotted / 'Ma died today,'" clearly an annual ritual. Douglas Dunn, mourning his late wife in "Anniversaries," writes that "each routine anniversary / At night, and noon, and dawn, / Are times I meet you, when souls rinse / Together in their moist reunions." He yearns for these meetings, and his anniversary fever goes beyond the typical she-was-born-on-this-date or she-died-on-that-date structure, extending to more routine matters at various moments throughout the day (*she went to bed at 10:00, so I'll keep going to bed at 10:00*).

Before my neurologist figured out the cause of my sudden onset of vertigo 355 days ago, my internist casually mentioned that he sees a lot of vertigo cases in the spring. Something about changes in weather and barometric pressure, maybe. So in the back of my mind, though I know spring wasn't the cause of my vertigo, I can't help noting that the equinox will arrive three days from now. Or that it's ten days before the first anniversary of Vertigo Day. All right, I know it's ridiculous, given the subsequent facts, for me to associate the coming of spring with another threat to my sense of balance. In his poem "Anniversaries," Thomas McGrath says, "anniversaries / Should have our praise, as trees / Salute the queenly coming of the Spring." Yes, yes, I could praise the coming anniversary as a milestone passed since I no longer have vertigo (KNOCK ON WOOD). But I still keep worrying that the Queen of Spring might again issue her order: *off with his head.*

I don't have many memories of my father because I didn't spend much time with him. He died when I was fourteen. For the three years before that, he'd been hospitalized, recovering from the crushing injuries to both legs sustained in a car accident. Before that, he'd always worked six days a week in the poultry market he owned, leaving home each morning by 5:00 and returning each evening at 7:00. Basically, I saw him on Sundays and for two hours on weekdays, times when he was exhausted and eager for me to be in another room. As a result of barely knowing or remembering him, I believe that I've sought to hold onto him through diligent, conscious observance of anniversaries. They provide a formal context to think and recall him at least twice a year, on his birth and death dates. To keep him alive in my brain and mind, present in my life's story, bringing back the time we rode a sled down a hill in Brooklyn's Prospect Park or the Saturday morning I spent with him at his market or the Sunday ball game at Ebbets Field when I watched his gnarled hands fumble with a miniature bottle of scotch. The anniversaries spur me to take out the old photo album with its half-dozen assorted images of him, to celebrate a *secret anniversary of the heart,* as Henry Wadsworth Longfellow says in his poem "Holidays": "the holiest of all holidays are those / Kept by ourselves in silence and apart; / The secret anniversaries of the heart, / When the full river of feeling overflows." They help me see him again, vivify him, though he has in truth all but vanished from me for good even as I draw closer to the place where he has gone.

I'm 62 years and 254 days old. In 351 days, I will have lived 10 years longer than my father, who died at age 53 and 239 days. On the other hand, it will take me 11,988 days to live as long as my mother, who was 95 years and 197 days old when she died. I never thought I'd live longer than my father did. Now I find myself trying to believe I'll catch my mother. This is a huge shift in perspective, from an anniversary-inspired vision of genetic doom to one of genetic blessing. Pessimism turning toward optimism as various anniversaries pass. Omens becoming milestones.

As I enter old age, I recognize that my anniversary fever induces a doubling of perspective. A delirium of timeposts, calendar mania. Not only am I driven to track anniversaries in compensation for earlier cognitive losses, and to use them as a springboard for all sorts of cockamamie computations, I'm now also doing what people my age naturally do: "It seems, as one becomes older, / That the past has another pattern, and ceases to be a mere sequence," as T. S. Eliot says in "The Dry Salvages." Looking back, noticing patterns, calculating, seeking a structure for both time and memory as time and memory run down, run out.

My brother, Philip, was buried the day I turned 50. He would have been 58 if he'd lived another 77 days. Late on the afternoon of my birthday, writing a note about the dates Philip had been born and died, I found myself remembering one of his great peeves: my bar mitzvah in 1960, celebrating the day I officially became a man according to religious law, had overshadowed his 21st birthday, celebrating the day he officially became a man according to secular law. Our parents, in consultation with the rabbi, had picked the date for my bar mitzvah, which was the day before Philip's birthday. The lavish party, the gifts, the recognition—the whole emphasis was on me instead of him. Now, freshly 50, I sat in my living room just before bedtime, grieving and looking at old photographs. And found myself chuckling, knowing that if he could, Philip would wink and say *I told you I'd get even.*

Holidays and days of special cultural significance seem to be when many significant events occur in my family life. My brother was born on September 11. He died on the Fourth of July. My father was born on Saint Patrick's Day, had his car accident on Columbus Day, and died on Veterans Day. The day of the viral attack on my brain was December 7, Pearl Harbor Day, the Day of Infamy. Good things can happen for me on holidays too: 18 years ago, Beverly and I first became lovers on Memorial Day. Some dates possess a peculiar familial synchronicity: my grandfather and my daughter were born on the same September date, 92 years apart; my great-grandfather arrived in his new home, America, on the same July date that Beverly and I moved into our new home here in Portland 106 years later; our May wedding date coincides with the 28th anniversary of my maternal grandmother's death. In a near-superfecta of temporal harmony, my wife and her mother, and my mother and *her* mother, were all born within eight days of one another.

In poetic tradition, love and anniversaries of love's touchstones have long possessed the power to stop time's erosion. Celebrating their first year together in "The Anniversary," John Donne assured his beloved that though "all kings, and all their favorites" and even "the sun itself" might be "elder by a year," and though "all other things to their destruction draw," nevertheless "only our love hath no decay." Love like theirs exists outside of time ("This, no tomorrow hath, nor yesterday"), forever young. Nearly 400 years later, Donald Justice makes the same point in "On an Anniversary," telling his wife that "thirty years and more go by / In the blinking of an eye, / And you are still the same." They have, in essence, tamed time: "Time joins us as a friend, / And the evening has no end." Of course neither Donne nor Justice believed this. They were operating within a romantic convention, one that may seem quaint in our current culture of irony and skepticism. But in September 2007, I found a blank journal I'd bought and never used. Its flyleaf was coffee stained, and between its first two pages, like a bookmark, was the receipt. It told me the name of the store on Fourth and Taylor in Portland, the Memorial Day purchase date from 15 years before, and the time: 3:07 p.m. So I knew the exact place and moment when I realized I was in love with Beverly. Because the journal, I remembered, was going to be the first one I'd ever kept, a record of dates and times and daily thoughts, a new approach where I would record regularly what was happening between us. But then I got back to my apartment that afternoon, set the journal aside while I prepared dinner for Beverly—who arrived after her day's work—and never did start journaling. The book, when I look at it now, seems to freeze the story of love at an instant full of hope and expectation, still asserting that anything can happen, that time stands still when lovers commit to each other. It's possible to see that the book, still all about hope and expectation, at once new and old, says something essential about the two of us together across all these years.

Each month after we first got together, I bought Beverly a small gift to commemorate the date. Earrings, a bracelet, a necklace. The game of Go, which we said we wanted to learn but never did. Over the course of 11 months, the process acquired its own momentum. I was in a serious flare-up of anniversary fever. Then, shortly before our one-year-of-being-together anniversary, Beverly and I married. She took over the management of our financial affairs, and, quite sensibly, suggested that the monthly gifts stop, since we now had another date to celebrate.

In his poem "Anniversaries," the British poet Douglas Dunn says "the calendar / Recurs to tell us who we are, / Or were." I've come to see that the marking of anniversaries has become vital to my sense of self. It connects me to a past that became fundamentally elusive when brain damage corrupted memory's function, and it affords me a feeling of stillness, even calm, amid the racing of events through time. It helps me to find order in a world that can be snarled and chaotic for anyone, not just for the brain damaged, or to find harmony in the jangle and dissonance of experience.

It's now two days after the first anniversary of Vertigo Day. I didn't have a sudden relapse. But I almost did. Two days ago Beverly and I were in an office located on the 27th floor of a new building on Portland's riverfront. As we approached its wall of windows, I swooned. My stomach and thighs felt like they did when I was a kid on a Coney Island Cyclone ride, weightless, plunging in freefall. I was dizzy in the same swirlingly helpless way that I'd been dizzy for

138 days last year. I didn't quite fall. Instead, I turned away and left the office. The elevator ride down turned my stomach again. For two hours I couldn't make the lightheadedness and queasiness stop. It was as if I'd unconsciously dared fate—how could I have done this on the anniversary!—and fate had responded with a cynical giggle.

Since I first read it 43 years ago, I've been haunted by W. S. Merwin's poem "For the Anniversary of My Death." Can anyone read it and not be? My memory is so poor that I can't recite any of my own poems by heart, but I can recite the first three lines of Merwin's: "Every year without knowing it I have passed the day / When the last fires will wave to me / And the silence will set out." I figure that this idea is the germ causing my anniversary fever. Track patterns all I want, read in them omens or milestones, distract myself from time's passage by focusing on the ways in which things keep coming back, I can't avoid the unknown anniversary that bookends my July birthday. The date when "I will no longer / Find myself in life" and my survivors will begin marking it.

Today is 136 days before the first anniversary of Vertigo Vanishing Day. It's one day less than 200 days before my mother's 100th birthday. It's 310 days before the first anniversary of the day my daughter's first book, *The Immortal Life of Henrietta Lacks*, was published. "Though time turns," Thomas McGrath says in "Anniversaries," "history moves / As if to prove our loves, / Having no pattern but the one we give."

Part Four

CARTWHEELS ON THE MOON

12

Elliptical Journey

When Beverly woke up I was standing a few feet from the end of our bed, naked, immobile, no longer shambling toward the bathroom. All my weight was on my right leg. My left hand probed my left hip.

"What're you doing?" she asked.

"Trying to figure out if I'm really awake."

I heard sheets rustle behind me, then the clack of eyeglasses snatched from the bedside table. "Is something wrong?"

"I think my hip just broke into a hundred pieces."

She got out of bed. This is something I always love to watch her do, but I couldn't turn around to see her. Couldn't put weight on my left hip, couldn't pivot or let the joint rotate in its socket. I doubted I'd ever move again. Which was ridiculous, and why I'd been considering my familiar it's-only-a-dream explanation.

"What happened?"

"I don't know. I got out of bed, took a couple of steps, and my hip exploded." I didn't think I'd done anything out of the ordinary. There'd been no warning something was about to go wrong, and the intense pain seemed worse for its suddenness. So at sixty-four, despite never having had a hip problem, despite lacking a diagnosis or even a hint of an explanation, my mind went right for the only obvious conclusion: *I need hip replacement. Today.* "I think this is a bad sign."

"Can you sit down?"

"I don't see how." With her help, I hopped backward on my right leg and sat on the bed's edge, but that hurt almost as much as walking had. None of this made sense. It was like there was a gap between *then* and *now* into which all the important information had fallen.

Beverly sat next to me. We looked at each other, not saying what we were both thinking: We're scheduled to leave for Spain in eight days. No way . . .

Throughout our first winter living downtown, Beverly and I had gone to the gym every other day. This was something new for us. We'd spent thirteen years living in the middle of twenty hilly acres of woods, our home a small isolated cedar yurt she'd built an hour southwest of Portland. For our daily walks we'd follow deer trails in a broad loop across the landscape, often accompanied by our three aged cats. Even in foul weather, sheltered by Douglas fir and the great limbs of old oak or wild cherry, we could be outside most days for a half hour of exercise, sometimes hacking overgrowth, sometimes wading through the risen creek.

I'd found the challenge of walking the woods to be more powerful than the hard five-mile runs I used to take daily in the years before getting sick in 1988. It took years of repetition before I could avoid getting lost if I could no longer see the house. But I loved these walks. They helped me regain some strength and balance. They helped me gain confidence that I could get around in the world, that I could find my way when things around (and within) me were confusing, fragmented, obscure. Walking like this wasn't just about exercise or regaining a modicum of fitness. It was about claiming my place again, too.

Now that we were in the heart of the city, living by the river, our daily exercise involved walking or riding bikes on the flat pathways along the water. All summer and fall, we'd kept company with osprey, herons, cormorants, ducks, gulls. We watched the swollen river recede from where it had overrun the bank and dwindle through the summer heat. Then cottonwood and ash on Ross Island, just across the river, lost their leaves and revealed a lagoon we'd been unable to see before. On one bike ride, a sassy Canada goose, turning quickly and hissing as I approached, made me skid and crash near the boat ramp at Willamette Park. But our ability to exercise was weather dependent. As winter neared, and we found ourselves exposed to the Northwest's heavy wind and rain, we realized the time had come to exercise indoors.

There was also a motive beyond maintaining fitness. We were planning a two-week trip in late spring that would involve some modest walking through the streets of Madrid, the hills of Andalucía, and—most ambitious—the steep elliptical core of Cuenca, built into the gorges above the Huécar and Júcar Rivers. So we wanted to prepare ourselves.

Oregon Health and Science University's Center for Health and Healing, just two blocks away from our new home, had a gym swarming with state-of-the-art fitness machines, free weights, cable equipment, mats, Pilates reformers, exercise balls. There were nooks and separate rooms for classes or consultations, blazing lights, mirrors everywhere. The place overlooked a shipbuilding yard, welders in their helmets at work amid a shower of sparks, giant blue cranes moving along their rails. There was so much going on, inside and out, that I found it hard to focus on what we were being told as we were led through the space. But we joined up, planning to work out there at our usual mellow pace while building up endurance and strength for Spain, and squeezing in river walks whenever the weather allowed.

Membership came with access to a personal trainer for two free sessions. Aaron's demeanor was gentle, his voice soft, everything about him suggesting that the gym was not going to be about intense, crazy muscle-building. He showed us how to use the equipment and helped us design moderate weight-lifting programs. Nothing here should be too hard for us. It was a gym, yes, but it was a health facility too, part of a medical institution. And, after all, I was nearing sixty-five, and had been disabled for more than a third of those years.

"Take it easy," he said, smiling, imagining—I suppose—that I would take heed.

Membership also came with a free T-shirt that said *Start where you are*. It was clear right away that I had no idea what this meant.

🌀

The old man rose and sank as though floating on air before the wall of windows.

He was well into his eighties, at least twenty years my senior, and worked the elliptical machine in slow motion, head cocked, towel draped around his neck, bald head lacquered with sweat. Earbud cords snaked from a pack at his waist. A single trek-pole lay on the floor beside his machine, within easy reach.

He'd been there when I arrived. I got on the machine next to him and snuck a look at its LCD display screen. His pace hovered around two miles per hour, then slowed and the machine thought the old man had quit so it flashed a message: PAUSE. EXIT WORKOUT? He carried on, bringing his workout session back online, and I began my own.

Until we enrolled at the gym, I'd never used an elliptical machine. But I'd heard all about its benefits, especially when compared with treadmills or road running. As the website Livestrong.com notes, the elliptical's primary advantage "is the reduction in stress on your hips, back and knees because your feet move with the machine and you don't have the pounding that comes with regular running." Used properly, it's designed to be a low-impact workout, equal parts cross-country skiing, stair climbing, treadmill running, and—with its modified cycling motion—stationary biking.

The elliptical machine is named for the motion of its pedals, the oval or closed-curve shape known in geometry as an ellipse. At the same time, you grip handrails that move back and forth as your legs pass through their elliptical rotation, so you look a little like you're smooth-dancing on a staircase or skating on foam. Theoretically, it's a versatile machine that exercises numerous muscle groups at once and provides strong cardiovascular work. Safe, easy on the joints, the skeleton. Just a few obvious precautions to note, such as to avoid standing on the balls of your feet or holding the handrails too hard or leaning forward or twisting your body as you stride. And as with any repetitive-motion activity, practice moderation because the most common elliptical machine injuries are due to overuse.

I hadn't been sure I could handle the machine's up-and-down-plus-back-and-forth motion without risking vertigo. I still couldn't handle heights or the multidirectional motion of a craft on water. But as long as I looked straight ahead and kept my eyes focused on an object, I could manage to maintain balance and avoid nausea.

Crazy as it sounds, working out near the old man kindled my competitive fire. But then, working out near anyone of any age, including Beverly as she used the treadmill, kindled my competitive fire. Equipment! Clocks and timers and stats! The machine's screen allowed me to view my exercise session as timed laps around a quarter-mile track, and I was riveted to the image as it traced my progress. Telling myself I wasn't concerned with anything but my own health, I couldn't stop glancing over to see how other exercisers were doing. What if my machine thought I'd quit my workout? If I was the only one in the gym, I'd have to outpace my last workout. By a lot. Despite the fact that I hadn't done anything more strenuous than those twenty-minute walks or half-hour bike rides with Beverly in the last two decades, once inside a gym, I couldn't help myself.

Any physician (as mine did), any trainer (as mine did), any sensible person (as Beverly did), even my T-shirt would warn me to take it easy. But despite recognizing that it would be bad for me, that I couldn't tolerate aerobic exercise in the aftermath of my illness, I couldn't listen to them. I knew better, after having been a serious long-distance runner in my thirties and forties, but the lure of working out was too powerful.

So I pushed myself during workouts on the elliptical, making sure my pace far exceeded the old man's. Sometimes, as I gripped the handrails and churned the pedals hard enough to feel myself struggling for balance, the idea would surface that this was absurd. No one else in the gym seemed to be nearing orbital velocity.

᭝

. . . . No way we're not going to Spain. Right? I mean, absolutely no way this trip gets canceled. We—and by We I mean Beverly—had worked so hard to plan and prepare for it. She'd taught herself Spanish, working for four months at her computer with a program called *Fluenz*. She'd figured out the impenetrable rules governing international cell phone and computer usage so that the telecommunications racket wouldn't bankrupt us as we used the web or kept in touch with people; as a backup, she'd learned how to use the experimental browser deep within Amazon's Kindle reader that allows for free Wi-Fi and 3G access to the Internet. She'd arranged accommodations that would cater to our gluten-free diet and satisfy our desire to spend time in small, out-of-the-way places, using her nascent Spanish—and sometimes Google Translate—to converse by phone or by e-mail with staff at Madrid hotels or in the mountains of Las Alpujarras. She'd booked flights; rented a car; set up the satellite navigation device; bought tickets so we could get into the Alhambra on the date and at the time that best suited us; ordered vests that had enough pockets and hidden compartments to safely carry whatever we might need, including—according to a dream I had—both of our wheeled suitcases. This was a trip for which endless contingencies had been considered and planned. And those plans had grown so complicated and mutually interconnected that the very idea of replicating this trip at some later date was mind-blowing. We will not cancel.

Therefore if I needed hip replacement surgery, I'd need the kind that let me recover full mobility and strength in about one week, including the ability to walk every day on hilly terrain. Meanwhile, Beverly relocated my old hazelwood cane so I could finally get to the bathroom.

When I spoke to my doctor a few minutes later, he wasn't optimistic. He told me there were several things that could cause the sort of sudden, immobilizing pain I'd described, and most of them weren't—as he put it—things I wanted to have. He sent me to the emergency room, calling ahead to be sure his friend the orthopedic surgeon would be aware of the case. And yes, he'd tell him that we needed to be on the fast track because of the trip to Spain, though I shouldn't get my hopes up.

But I'm all about high hopes, especially in inverse proportion to their probability. In 1988 and 1989, the early days of my illness when I was bedbound and unable to read or write or maintain balance, I never doubted I would find a way back. Not fully back, I understood that, but back to some level of meaningful function. As Viktor E. Frankl said in *The Doctor and the Soul*, "Man must cultivate the flexibility to swing over to another value-group if that group and that alone offers the possibility of actualizing values. Life requires of man spiritual elasticity, so that he may temper his efforts to the chances that are offered." Neurological damage had thrown me out of the value-group where I'd wanted to be—I could no longer think or remember or move as I had, could no longer succeed in the ways that I valued—so I had to find another value-group, one based on a realistic understanding of my capacities. From where I was then, it was a triumph just to write a coherent sentence, just to remember the name of a person I'd met or my new phone number when Beverly and I got together, just to walk—with my cane—up to the mailbox and back. The worse things are for me, the more optimistic I become. It's when things are going well that I worry most.

So as we approached Good Samaritan Hospital on the morning of May 17, I was feeling certain we'd be arriving in Madrid on the morning of May 26 as planned. I left the emergency room five hours later with aluminum crutches, a prescription for Percocet, and a recommendation to see the orthopedic surgeon the next day. Beverly made the appointment by cell phone, as we left the hospital. I'd had a shot of the nonsteroidal anti-inflammatory drug Toradol, which slightly mellowed the pain. I'd also had X-rays and a CT scan, and the attending physician thought there might be evidence of a fracture in the hip along with something he called calcific tendinopathy. He couldn't make a definitive diagnosis, but the surgeon would have the results by the time of my appointment the next afternoon.

※

"Beverly!" A woman screamed my wife's name and semaphored from across the waiting room. She rushed over to us. "It's me," she said, grabbing Beverly's hands, "remember?"

Clearly not. Smiling, reflecting back this woman's delight, Beverly tried to place the face and voice, and in that space when past and present poised before us, time seemed to stop. I knew what it felt like to be there, unable to recall, to make experience cohere. Memory may be the ultimate elliptical narrative, compressed, tersely expressed, built around great gaps in the flow of time and information. With so much missing, it's essentially ambiguous, packed with symbols, suggestive, open to interpretation, pruned of the superfluous even when some of what we recall seems trivial. And it's fluid, varying and evolving through the years. Yet we long for certainty, clarity—in our memories, of course, but in most of our immediate experience as well. We want coherence in the moment. I have to know what's wrong with my hip. I need a story that links what I've done in the past with what has brought me to a halt now. But even in medical science, in the diagnosis and treatment of injury, ambiguities dominate. I'm not as tolerant of this as I'd like to be, or as I've imagined myself after all these years of daily experience with cognitive fragmentation.

The woman, who managed the surgeon's office, turned out to be one of Beverly's long-lost best friends from high school. When she said her name, I could see time begin its usual flow again for Beverly. It was clear that her friend had sharp recall of events that Beverly had forgotten until hearing about them now, and there was a kind of relief in the way the story expanded. *The Baskin-Robbins Store Escapade! The Clandestine Drives Out to the Airport.*

She escorted us to an exam room and said she'd be surprised if I still needed the crutches when the appointment was over. Before I could figure out what that might imply, a physician's assistant arrived, burly, full of energy, clearly no stranger to gyms and workouts. He heard my story, read my paperwork, looked at the radiologist's report, poked around my hip. Nah, no fracture, no tendinopathy. I had trochanteric bursitis, a repetitive stress injury to the point of the hip almost certainly brought about by overuse, repetitive motion, and aging, and distinguished by just this sort of sharp, intense, localized pain. The small, jellyish sac that's supposed to cushion a joint's bones from the soft overlying tissue had become inflamed. Surgery wasn't necessary.

"I'll shoot you," he said, and left the room.

He returned with a kit that scared the bejeezus out of me, a long and thick-needled syringe filled with corticosteroids and analgesics that required ample time and internal maneuvering to empty into my hip. I heard Beverly's indrawn breath as the procedure began. And, though limping and glad I'd taken a Percocet a couple hours before the appointment, I did walk out of the office without relying on my crutches.

🌀

The hiccups began late the next morning and lasted ten hours. I'd sip a cup of water, they'd stop, I'd relax a few minutes, and they'd resume. I couldn't figure out what was causing them, and kept recalling the terrifying 1958 news story, when I was eleven, about Pope Pius XII dying of hiccups. Of course, his lasted off and on for five years, but still . . .

Beverly was the one who thought of the possible connection between my hiccups and the corticosteroid shot. Then she checked the Internet, where it was confirmed by articles in such journals as *Anesthesia & Analgesia* or *Neuroendocrinology Letters*, which states that "hiccups occurring secondary to high doses of corticosteroids are a well-recognized problem." I was fortunate to have only ten hours' worth since, according to several online discussion groups, they often last for days.

My hot flashes began the morning after the hiccups. Over the course of about an hour, my face and neck and chest flushed scarlet, crimson, carmine. I couldn't cool down, couldn't stop sweating. I sat on the couch fanning myself with a rolled-up sports section from the

Oregonian and sighing as I flickered reds like a neon sign. Beverly tried very hard not to gloat. *Now you know what I went through.* Back on the Internet, she found confirmation of the hot flash/steroids connection. *OMG!* someone had written in a discussion thread. *Both of my hands and halfway up my forearms are blushed!*

But the hip pain was almost entirely gone in a couple of days, fading steadily after that except when I slept on it too long or, especially, if I put too much stress on it. But I would never do something like that.

Beverly and I resumed walking outdoors as the May weather softened, testing the hip, trying to build up my confidence for the last few days before our trip would begin. The only lingering issue was a deadened feeling deep in the joint, a sense of disconnection, as though my hip were not quite mine, or not quite participating in our activities.

As Beverly and I packed, I wondered about bringing along my cane. Just in case. I didn't need anything extra to carry, that's for sure, but I was worried about what would happen if the pain returned, if something caused the bursa to re-inflame. And having a cane did make it possible to board flights early and therefore secure the overhead storage space. No, I was okay, I was going to be okay. Cane-less.

§

And I was okay until Cuenca, seven days into our travels. Looking back through my journal, I'm astounded to see how much we walked. On the evening of our arrival, awake for nearly twenty-four hours and searching for one of the many tapas bars that allegedly served gluten-free items, we wandered from our hotel in central Madrid to the Plaza del Sol, crammed with political demonstrators, and back, a two-hour concrete ramble. In Andalucía we walked whitewashed villages and hill towns in the foothills of La Subbética, walked the dog named Ruby who lived at the olive farm where we were staying, walked through the entire religious heart of Córdoba from the Great Mosque to the fourteenth-century synagogue in the old Jewish quarter, and walked the grounds of the Alhambra and the steep hill down through the maze of the ancient Albayzín in Granada. Only eight days earlier it was impossible to imagine that I could've walked this much, even on flat terrain at a moderate pace and with frequent coffee breaks. Yet my journal makes no mention of hip pain until Cuenca.

Cuenca looked like what it was: an elliptically shaped, hilltop fortress town constructed by eighth-century Moors on a ridge above two river gorges. Its *Casas Colgadas*, or hanging houses, are built into the sheer rock wall and have perched over the Huécar gorge for six hundred years. The entire Old Town was up there on the hill, and nearly devoid of level walking surfaces, a labyrinth of twisting and crisscrossing lanes and worn staircases. New Town, built well after Cuenca's need to serve as a fortress, was located down by the river, nearly a hundred fifty feet below.

Beverly and I stayed in the Parador, a converted convent located across the gorge and connected to Cuenca's upper reaches by the narrow, low-railed St. Paul Bridge. One look unfortunately brought to my mind the Peruvian span that broke and "precipitated five travelers into the gulf below" in Thornton Wilder's tragic 1927 novel, *The Bridge of San Luis Rey*.

After we checked in, Beverly sat in our room's window seat overlooking the bridge and hanging houses, plotting out our walk. First, we'd cross the bridge, thereby allowing me a definitive triumph over vertigo, then explore Old Town. Next morning, we'd walk downhill from the Parador and cross the river at ground level to explore New Town, then wind our way up to the abstract art and contemporary art museums of Old Town that had been closed the night before, and cross the bridge at day's end.

The bridge crossing went well. I walked about four steps behind Beverly and never stopped looking at her lovely butt, even when she paused to take a photo of the hanging houses in the dusky light. By the time we reached the far side, I was giddy with the success of my crossing. But the relentless hill walking began to wear me down, and I needed to take half a Percocet before I felt comfortable enough to sleep. Which should have been adequate warning that I was in the same sort of overuse zone that I'd frequented when churning away in the gym.

I finally made the connection the next day, while sitting on the plaza outside Los Arcos, the same Basque restaurant where we'd eaten the night before. We'd done our walk, descending one hundred fifty feet and working our way back up, and my hip felt both dead and tortured at once. Still under the illusion that I had things under control, I'd asked the waiter at Los Arcos to bring me "un copa cappuccino" instead of "un tazo cappuccino" and therefore was sipping a wine glass–sized espresso drink. In the ninety-degree heat, sore and abashed, I thought about the week ahead, including six days walking around Madrid with my daughter and her boyfriend, and realized I'd come full circle, or rather full ellipsis. It was me and the old man, again, only now I recognized that I was the old man too. I'd been working out with the wrong goals in mind—I shouldn't have been trying to beat him, I should have been trying to emulate him. Work each day at the proper capacity so I could keep going, continually monitoring and adjusting my goals, staying strong enough and balanced enough to keep on getting stronger and more balanced.

I smiled at Beverly, and we got up to pay for my vat of cappuccino, half-empty on the table. We went back to the Parador, crossing the bridge side by side and hand in hand, for a long afternoon nap. Not even the caffeine in my system could keep me awake.

෧

The old man is floating in front of the windows again. It's almost a month since I last saw him, and as I approach the array of machines I find myself stopping to watch him. He looks calm, his expression only a few degrees shy of a smile, and he seems to be looking at the hull of a barge taking shape in the shipyard across the way.

I'm not going to get back on an elliptical machine. This hadn't really become clear to me until just this moment. I know that my hip injury wasn't so much about the machine as about my behavior on it. But still, that flattened circle gait, that elliptical rotation, is a strange motion, at least for me. Why tempt fate? The hip feels okay.

Beverly gets on a treadmill and turns back to look at me before starting her workout. She raises her eyebrows and moves her hand in a small arc, inviting me onto the treadmill machine next to her. When I begin my routine, I force myself not to look at her display screen. Or at the old man afloat three machines to the right.

13

To Land's End and Back

A 1,512-Mile Drive

Around Southern England

The British exaggerate when they call this a road. It's at best a roadlet, a paved path. Something roadish. Across a fold of the map, and in my dreams for the next month, it has a four-digit, B-road number too blurred to decipher. Call it B-XXX.

I see B-XXX bend west two hundred yards ahead. There are no road signs and I can't detect the change sooner because high hedgerows and overhanging trees obscure my view, further narrowing the absurdly tight space, creating shadowy blocks, distorting perspective. Then a burly black van bursts through the curve and speeds straight at us.

My instinct is to jerk the wheel left. But I know—have been repeating to myself like a mantra, even before Beverly started saying it—that there's *a stone wall to the left*, completely camouflaged within foliage. We're as far over there as we can dare to go, but still seem to take up more than half the road. There's no center stripe. It's like hurtling along a bobsled run and meeting sudden oncoming traffic. I tap the brake, not wanting to risk a swerve, and hold the wheel hard as our car shudders in the van's passing. My side-view mirror is blasted flat against the door. I don't know how we survive.

"Did you see how close that was?" I ask Beverly.

"I just shut my eyes."

We're silent for a moment. She checks the map and makes an adjustment to our GPS device, which responds by announcing that it's recalculating. Which is what Beverly and I are doing too, recalculating the dimensions of our latest hair's-breadth escape on British roads. This one isn't quite as horrifying as when I ran over some sort of mound cloaked at a road's edge and almost flipped the car while eluding a caravan near Land's End, or when the left-front tire smashed across a hidden boulder in a remote corner of western Cornwall. But with its nightmarishly darkened, pinched setting and video-game intensity, and with its apparent normalness as a British driving experience—its modest ordinariness—the encounter on B-XXX is emblematic.

We'd come to Great Britain for two weeks of scenic touring. Just the south and southwest of the island this time, seeing landscape and gardens and stone circles, paying homage at a few literary sites. We'd take walks in the Cotswolds and on Bodmin Moor, along Carmarthen Bay, in Dorset and Cornwall, where we'd also have a picnic at Land's End. There was so much we wanted to see. Beverly had lived in Great Britain for four years in the early 1980s, and I had been there in 1969, when I was twenty-two. We loved the Great Britain we remembered, loved the art and literature, the land, the history, and wanted to see it together. But we didn't want to overschedule our vacation or put ourselves in a time bind. So Beverly sacrificed visits to the grounds of Blenheim Palace, landscaped by Capability Brown, and to the gardens of Barnsley House or the Rollright stones from the Bronze Age, and I chose Thomas Hardy and Dylan Thomas over T. S. Eliot or the Dymock poets, and skipped a stop at the Hay-on-Wye bookstores. Eliot, whose *Four Quartets* I loved, was particularly hard for me to skip. I'd started researching where the sites that had inspired individual Quartets were located, saw that Burnt Norton and East Coker were not too far from where we planned to be, and stopped before checking out Little Gidding, telling myself that we'd be back in England again, and I could catch up with Eliot then. *What might have been is an abstraction / Remaining a perpetual possibility.*

I'd anticipated that there might be some narrow roads here and there, and had noted Paul Theroux's comment, in *The Kingdom by the Sea*, that "driving on English roads was no fun." But the B-roads, farm roads, byways, and single-tracks were proving to be far more perilous than I'd imagined. So were a lot of the so-called A-roads. Maybe we needed to rethink our strategy for seeing what we wanted to see while not dying.

When the next oncoming vehicle appears on a long B-XXX straightaway, I have just enough time to stop and back up toward a slight wrinkle in the shoulder I'd noticed moments earlier. Even tucked into it, I'm not sure the accelerating blood-red Saab will make it past us.

§

Within two hours of renting a car, I realized that the true challenge wouldn't be what I'd expected: driving on the wrong side of the road, with the steering wheel on the wrong side of the car and the stick shift on the wrong side of the steering wheel. Those wonderlandy, mirror-world British elements required concentration and practice, and never did become second nature, yet were manageable right away. But the roads! So many brought to mind the ancient foot or cart paths they may once have been. Think of the occasional country lane in the United States where only one car at a time can cross a narrow old bridge; then think of that road stretching for dozens of twisty miles with two-way traffic and a speed limit of sixty miles an hour; then imagine it so overgrown that everything beyond and within it was hidden, or like a tight tunnel open (sometimes) to a bit of sky. Then picture it littered and bordered with potholes and obstacles that slashed tires, walloped rims, jolted chassis.

And it wasn't just a matter of the back roads. In towns, already-narrow streets were further crimped by cars or vans or delivery vehicles parked half-on and half-off sidewalks. Some streets dead-ended without warning or room to turn around. There were high curbs ideally designed to hammer tires, and, when traffic could pass in only one direction at a time, a system of unspecified protocols ensuring that you could proceed only when oncoming vehicles were likely to force you curbside.

Road signs presented vast amounts of irrelevant or ambiguous information, as though Monty Python had been in charge of their design. *The Bureau of Silly Signs.* Newspapers routinely featured stories about driver confusion: Crossroads where dozens of signs clustered just a few hundred feet from the turn, a cascade of information about speed limits, nearby attractions, distances, cautions, permanent and temporary prohibitions, instructions. According to the *Daily Mail*, "At one junction near Oldham, motorists are told not to turn left, not to turn right, to give way and to keep to the 40mph speed limit— all at the same time." Some signs contained a red circle with a line through a prohibited activity while others, also prohibitive, contained a red circle without a line. Arrows indicating that a road turns left might appear where the road turns right. A sign known affectionately as "the Evel Knievel Sign" seemed to show a motorbike vaulting over an automobile. While meant to indicate that no motor vehicles are allowed on the road, it could as easily be construed to mean that motorbikes have the right-of-way or that motorbike stunts are forbidden. A recent survey of 524 drivers showed that none could understand all twelve signs they were shown, and only one-fourth managed to identify half of them. I thought we might be safer just to ignore signs altogether, but on a road in Dorset, we passed several signs that said SUDDEN GUNFIRE.

When told by his readers that "trying to drive in Great Britain and Ireland was a nerve-wracking and regrettable mistake," travel writer Rick Steves advised them to "adjust your perceptions of personal space." As though the problem were one of attitude or manners, solvable by a tweak of perspective. He added, "It's not 'my side of the road' or 'your side of the road.' It's just 'the road.'" Sage-sounding advice, except Steves failed to mention that the road, "shared as a cooperative adventure" (!), is actually an arena of temporal-spatial pandemonium in which space age automobile technology meets medieval road design and neolithic human combat impulses.

🌀

Out of necessity, Beverly and I became avid students of the British road classification system. First, there were letter codes: M-roads, the motorways radiating out from London, were like American freeways; A-roads were the main routes between towns; B-roads were secondary routes; and then there were unclassified roads. But the letters didn't tell you much about road size or condition, and we'd driven A-roads that were narrower and more treacherous than some B-roads. The secret—the mystery—was in the number of digits that followed those letters. More digits meant the road was more remote and usually smaller. Some three-digit roads and most four-digit roads—the roads we most wanted to drive on to get to the places we most wanted to go—were roadlets.

Beverly, our navigator, studied maps and worked on the GPS device, which had its own struggle with the roads, their twists and habit of vanishing into one another, their tendency to shrink toward tracks. The device, whose voice we named Emma, kept thinking we were in the middle of fields rather than on roads, an understandable confusion. *Turn left! Then turn left again!* In our rooms and our car, folding and refolding maps, programming and reprogramming Emma, Beverly was a genius at estimating dimensions and likely visibility and potential traffic flow for various routes, but still sometimes had to revise them in a flash, according to conditions on the ground. Meanwhile, I tried to keep us on the roads' surfaces and out of fields.

In February, three months before our trip, we'd reserved a Ford Focus, opting for a car roughly the same size and shape, and with a similar range of driver visibility, as our seven-year-old Honda CR-V. But when we got to the Avis counter at Heathrow, the rental agent was very persuasive. He'd just received a shipment of new 2012 Alfa Romeo Giuliettas, and he could give us one for only a little more than the Ford would cost. But since we planned to drive so much, and the Giulietta used diesel fuel, and the price of gas was so high in Great Britain, we'd end up saving a lot of money while having the pleasure of two weeks in such a sharp vehicle.

That all made sense while we were standing there going over the figures, and it made sense when I saw the snazzy red car itself, the sort of sporty thing I'd never driven before (six gears to shift through with my left hand while remembering that turning right meant crossing oncoming traffic and that when I entered a roundabout, I had to drive left). Of course, under the circumstances I should have understood that never having driven such a car before was a drawback, not an attraction.

As we headed toward Oxford, our destination for the first two days, I was confused about why the Giulietta felt so large since it was actually smaller than our Honda. It was shorter in height by eight and a half inches and in length by ten inches, and was a half inch narrower. But together these dimensions meant that the Giulietta put me closer to the ground than I was used to. At the same time, because it was configured with a long snout and chunky rear, a lot more of the car was in front of me than I was used to. It seemed huge out there, like I was steering a limousine; its hood bulged to accommodate an aerodynamic crease in its design; and I'm only five foot four. All this combined to limit my visibility over the Giulietta's front edges and down to the road. I struggled to keep from hitting the left front tire against curbs when I parked or was forced close to the road's edge.

※

If we followed B-roads most of the way it would take ninety minutes to drive the forty miles from Hidcote Manor Garden back to Oxford. It had already been a long day. Wanting to finish a three-hour walk in the Cotswold Hills before the weather got too hot or the hills crowded, we'd left Oxford early and taken A-40, a broad divided highway where my main problem was remembering that the left lane was the slow lane. Exiting at Burford, we looped through a series of narrowing roads with widening route numbers toward the River Eye in the village of Lower Slaughter, where we planned to start our walk. A friend back in Oregon had told us that following the Warden's Way from Lower to Upper Slaughter and beyond was like dropping into a Jane Austen novel, and a 2011 Google Streetview Poll had named Lower Slaughter's Copse Hill Road "the Most Romantic Street in Britain." Even so, after a few minutes we could tell that paved road, with its view of sprawling estates and the occasional vehicle forcing us to step aside, wasn't what we were after. We could experience *that* while driving. So we returned to our car to figure out an alternative site for our walk.

As Beverly studied her maps and notes, I sat passing the ignition key from hand to hand and realized that for the last two days—ever since renting the car—I'd been paying inadequate attention to where we actually were. I loved seeing the landscape and villages we passed, but had been so focused on the roads and the management of the Giulietta, on the crazy driving conditions and the still-awkward shifting of gears and the car's endless alarms about roadside traffic cameras and the stay-on-the-left business, that I had little sense of specific places, the flow of geography, what was near what, or which roads we'd been on at any moment. I was missing Great Britain, except in the most general way, except as a kind of slide show. Lines from *Four Quartets* came to mind while I closed my eyes, stretched, and waited for Beverly's instructions: *I am here or there, or elsewhere*, from "East Coker," and *I can only say* there *we have been: but I cannot say where*, from "Burnt Norton." Then, when I glanced over at Beverly, more lines from "East Coker": *Love is most nearly itself when here and now cease to matter*. It was as though Eliot had determined to offer appropriate commentary and mystical guidance in counterpoint to Emma's practical GPS advice, insisting that there was indeed room for him on this trip after all. Move over, Hardy and Thomas.

While I was dealing with Eliot, Beverly had mapped out a route along B-4077 and a slinky unnumbered lane to the village of Stanton, where we could access a long, circular walk on the Cotswold Way National Trail. All her research was paying off. She knew exactly where we were and what was near what, and she had backup plans ready in case things didn't work out.

Just outside the Slaughters we stopped for Beverly to photograph a blooming rapeseed field, and as I watched I became aware of how tight my neck and shoulder muscles were, the result of a constantly tensed back and a left arm unused to all the repetitive shifting of gears. Early symptoms of B-road Syndrome. I needed to focus on the right things, and avoid transforming the journey into one extended driving test. I remembered Eliot's lines from "Little Gidding," which struck me now as ominous: *What you thought you came for is only a shell, a husk of meaning.* No, Mr. Eliot, I knew what I came for was rich with meaning, especially if I let myself find it.

A half hour later, we parked in the Parish Council lot beside Stanton's cricket grounds. Chatter, cheers, and the pock of a solid hit drew me over to the fence for a closer look at the game, and we stayed long enough to watch a white-clad batsman slug a ball into what would be deep left on a baseball field. Then we followed Cotswold Way signposts through the village, past a thatched cottage and small pond, and began the steep climb through tall beech trees that seemed to lead us out of time. The morning was now emphatically quiet except for the sound of our feet in the grass and our breathing. Hard as the going was, I could feel myself relax and my muscles begin to find balance. We stepped over a few stiles and out into sunlight just beyond the kissing gate. As I looked back, I saw we were alone. The view rolled east toward Snowshill and I could see no evidence of cars anywhere. For three hours, I didn't think about driving at all.

Hungry after our walk, we skipped the backroads and took A-44 straight to Moreton-in-Marsh. For three months, ever since Beverly had found out about Mrs. T. Potts Tea Room online, we'd been anticipating their Cream Tea with homemade gluten-free scones. They even had a gluten-free version of leek and cheese quiche. We saved room for the scones, and when they arrived I tore one open. Beverly gasped and said, "No way that's gluten-free, it's too fluffy and sticky." We called to the owner, who also gasped. The waitress had brought out the wrong scones, and the owner replaced them for us gratis. It was hard to tell if this sequence of events was good or bad. I heard Eliot say, *It was not what one had expected.*

We walked the old market town's High Street picking up supplies for a light picnic dinner back in Oxford. Then we drove eleven slow miles, some of them along the ancient Fosse Way dating back to Roman days, to Hidcote Manor Garden. A pigeon greeted us—*the bird called, in response to the unheard music hidden in the shrubbery*—as we entered Hidcote's series of small gardens conceived as distinct thematic rooms—a white room, a red room, a room containing a circular pool—with hedges, hornbeam, and yew trees as walls separating each room. We tried to appreciate the plan that Lawrence Johnston had come up with for his garden, but even though we were outside, and had occasional panoramic views across the Vale of Evesham, it felt like we were in a big, rambling mansion, its individual rooms lavish and eye-catching but random, lacking flow, lacking a sense of wholeness. And to me, the flowers *had the look of flowers that are looked at.*

We were tired as we left Hidcote, but not in a hurry to get back to Oxford. Beverly was taking landscape photographs to inspire her painting when she returned to her studio, and I was reveling in Eliot's company, wanting to stay out longer to see what he might say next, concerned that he might go away once we stopped our day's travels. I was also feeling more confident about driving. So we decided to stick with our plans and follow the B-roads back to Oxford.

Just over two miles later, as cramped Hidcote Road led us through the village of Ebrington, I glanced to my right and saw an oval sign on the stone wall at the entrance of a driveway. It said *Little Gidding.*

I braked and pulled over to the left, hitting the front tire on the curb—something I hadn't done all day—and sat with both hands on the wheel, unwilling to believe I'd accidentally driven right to the place that had inspired Eliot's final Quartet. That would simply be too weird. I hadn't realized we were anywhere near it. And I thought I was about to cry.

"What happened?" Beverly asked.

"Oh my God."

I felt overcome by a profound feeling of revelation, one of those *timeless moments* that Eliot wrote about throughout the Quartets, an understanding that I was being led to the places where I most needed to be. It didn't matter what I came here for, only what I found. Or what found me. *The purpose is beyond the end you figured and is altered in fulfillment.* Despite all that I'd been allowing to distract me, the power of this moment—discovering myself at Little Gidding as though drawn there—put me in deep contact with the spirit of Eliot's poem, its search for the miraculous in the everyday. *Here the impossible union of spheres of existence is actual.* Poetry itself was alive in me and in the world, working an unexpected magic. Having decided I did not have time on this trip to see the places that inspired Eliot's Quartets, poems so saturating my memory that lines returned almost on their own, unbidden, I was nonetheless led directly to one of those places, without knowing quite where it was or where I was in relation to it. *In order to arrive at what you do not know you must go by a way which is the way of ignorance.* The experience was transcendent, both timeless and immediate, exactly the sort of thing that travel should provide.

ⓢ

One reason I hadn't realized we were anywhere near Little Gidding as we drove through Ebrington was that we weren't anywhere near Little Gidding as we drove through Ebrington. At least, not the Little Gidding that inspired Eliot's poem.

As I discovered later, the Little Gidding we'd passed was actually a cozy bed-and-breakfast offering two guest suites and a private lounge. A stone house set far back off the road, it had been built and operated by two elderly women who felt that an orchard site they were purchasing, with its air of peace and tranquility, and its pigs rooting among the trees (*leave the rough road and turn behind the pig-sty*), reminded them of the place Eliot had written about, so they named it Little Gidding. It was an homage—in name only—and far from the real thing.

Had I thought about it clearly, had the details behind Eliot's poem remained more present for me than its music and themes and a scattering of its lines, had I studied it rather than simply savored its lyrical pleasures, I might have remembered that he'd written about a settlement—a former Anglican religious community—and its chapel, located in Huntingdonshire, ninety miles northeast of Ebrington. But in the moment, tired, distracted, dodging around and between parked and oncoming cars, tense behind the wheel, B-road crazy, I responded to the sign Little Gidding with pure emotion. I was there! I'd been visited by the miraculous.

In "The Dry Salvages," the Quartet preceding "Little Gidding," Eliot wrote about certain *moments of happiness* or *of sudden illumination* that we come to understand only much later. He says *We had the experience but missed the meaning.* In Ebrington, encountering a Little Gidding, an out-of-the-way bed-and-breakfast in a remote corner of the North Cotswolds near Chipping Campden, but believing that I'd been led to Eliot's community of Little Gidding with its rebuilt seventeenth-century retreat and famous church, I *had the meaning but missed the experience.*

It didn't occur to me to research Little Gidding online when we got back to Oxford. I knew I'd eventually get around to that, imagining I'd write an essay back home about the literary sites I'd visited. I was content just to savor what had happened.

The delusion lasted until the following evening. First, we drove five hours—most of them on highways luxuriant with lanes—to Llandeilo, in southern Wales. We arrived at our hotel just before two, still in time for its massive Sunday lunch, then napped and woke to find a blue-and-purple-striped hot-air balloon descending toward a field across the road and lifting off again in the late afternoon light. Seeing its slow gentle movements, hearing the occasional soft whoosh of its burner firing, feeling a little groggy from sleep and relaxed by the first easy day of driving since we'd begun the tour, I decided to phone my daughter in Chicago and tell her about our astonishing rendezvous with Little Gidding.

Rebecca was excited for me, sharing my astonishment over what had happened and what was to come. Unlike me, though, she responded to astonishment by asking for facts. Where exactly was the Eliot site I'd stumbled on? What kind of place was it? She encouraged me to write everything down, send her occasional travel notes if I wished, and followed up with an e-mail asking for more detail. Anticipating that I would want to write about my upcoming visit to Hardy country, she urged me to track down my lost college honors thesis on his novels, something I never would have thought to do. I wanted to write back immediately, but realized I was uncertain about exactly where we'd seen Little Gidding. I also realized that I couldn't remember much about what had so inspired Eliot, what Little Gidding actually was or what it meant to him. So first Beverly retraced for me the route we'd taken from Hidcote. Ebrington! Then, as I wrote an e-mail to Rebecca, Beverly Googled Little Gidding and began to read about it.

"Oh," she said, passing me the laptop. "Take a look at this."

A few minutes later, I changed the subject line of my e-mail to "Uh, the wrong Little Gidding."

※

After that, Eliot's voice faded, replaced by the racket of Dylan Thomas as we drove around Carmarthenshire and into the Black Mountains. At Thomas's boathouse in Laugharne, approaching nearby Sir John's Hill, or walking the shore and cliffs at Pendine, it was possible to imagine him, at least for moments, in touch with a sober and genuine ecstasy. *I open the leaves of the water at a passage of psalms and shadows.* That feeling stayed with me when Beverly and I visited the National Botanic Garden and drove in the Brecon Beacons

National Park, as we climbed into the ruins of Dinefwr Castle and walked its Dragonfly Trail in late afternoon. For a few days, I'd had no nightmares about cars careening toward ours in the depths of long tunnels or about a massive truck appearing suddenly before me as the road funneled us into its maw. I was, I believed, gaining ease with the driving situation, had begun to find what Thomas called *fountain in the weather of fireworks, Cathedral calm*. Maybe driving hadn't been quite as bad as it seemed last week.

By the time we left Wales and headed to Cornwall, I'd begun to convince myself that road size and conditions, road signs, roadside obstacles, or daredevil drivers were problems I could handle through skeptical scrutiny and flexibility. Ease up, Floyd, it's not as bad as you make it seem. It felt liberating to consider that our journey was all about improvisation, that route recommendations—whether provided by the GPS, hotel staff or guests, or guidebooks—couldn't be trusted, and that maps lied, their determination that a road was scenic seeming to ignore the presence of high, view-canceling hedgerows or knotty curves. One evening in Wales, we decided to visit Carreg Cennen Castle, a thirteenth-century ruin visible from various roads near our hotel. Located just four and a half miles southeast of Llandeilo, it took forty-five minutes to reach on the steep, winding, one-lane, roundabout roads by which Emma directed us, and we arrived just as the castle and its park closed for the night. We might have gotten there a few minutes earlier if one of the roads hadn't been a dead end so narrow that I couldn't turn around in it, and had to back sinuously out of for nearly a half mile. At the park gate, the departing supervisor described a route to Llandeilo that took us back in ten minutes. It was possible, I supposed, to laugh about that.

Then we went to Cornwall. After four days of driving around the region, we knew we had to avoid B-roads for the remaining three days of our travels. Even before Cornwall, the left front tire and wheel rim were scraped and scuffed from encounters with curbs. We were concerned that we'd have to pay for a replacement tire. So when B-3315 south of St. Ives couldn't contain both the Giulietta and an oncoming caravan, and I was forced so far left that we nearly flipped as the wheels passed over a hidden bank of dirt, we were relieved that there was no further damage to the vehicle. But later that afternoon, heading back north on a slender vein of B-3315 near Penzance, when a gleaming black Land Rover suddenly filled the road, I veered away and smashed the same left front tire across a boulder jutting from the bottom of the hedgerow. The force was so great, the jarring so thorough, and the sound so loud, we were sure the car's chassis or body had been mangled or the wheel destroyed. I pulled over and we got out to assess the damage. The impact had been confined to the tire and wheel, but the rubber was now profoundly gouged in two places, with flaps like torn skin revealing the inner tire wall. Beverly tried to nudge the flaps back in place but we knew they weren't likely to stay. The wheel's rim was dented and marred, shabby rather than sporty.

We looked at each other, grateful to have escaped worse harm, understanding that we had to avoid any further contact between that tire and an obstacle. From now on, we'd stick to the dual carriageways and main roads as much as possible, inspect the tire and gauge its pressure every time we got out of the car, worry over every bump.

⟳

We drove southeast to Dorset almost entirely on A-38 and A-35, fat trunk roads with only two digits to their name, true highways. Once there, we didn't have to drive much because we'd planned to spend time on foot. We walked a windy, cold half mile from our B&B to Lulworth Cove, "the small basin of sea" where Sergeant Francis Troy staged his disappearance in *Far from the Madding Crowd*. Later in the evening, we walked the Weymouth shoreline. In and around

Dorchester the next morning, we explored the town's heart, where *The Mayor of Casterbridge* had been set and where the county museum had a vast exhibit of Hardy-related material. We spent over an hour at his Max Gate home and strolled the nut walk, *the alley of bending boughs* Hardy had planted himself. We walked a long wooded path over the heath at his birthplace in Higher Bockhampton, and spent an hour at his grave in Stinsford churchyard.

Going to a small pub that catered to gluten-free diets, we followed a road through the Lulworth Firing Range, a Ministry of Defense zone normally closed to traffic. It was open now in honor of the Queen's Diamond Jubilee holidays, but few tourists seemed to know. We drove on an ancient ridge road, its view toward Dorset's Jurassic Coast clear and panoramic, and as I came out of a blind curve a dozen shaggy sheep were spread across the road. I braked, thinking that after all I'd done to the tire it would be a perfect cartoon ending for a flock of sheep to cause the blowout.

In late afternoon, and at the advice of our host, we crossed the road and began walking a mile across Hambury Tout. This large chalk hill leads toward the coast and Durdle Door, a natural lime-stone arch cut by the sea, which draws a quarter-million tourists a year. As on our walk in the Cotswolds, we found ourselves alone in the countryside. But then, as we crested Hambury Tout, we saw that the Coastal Path was covered by hundreds of tourists. Some were standing on a platform above Durdle Door, some were marching like pilgrims east toward Lulworth Cove or west toward Weymouth. Foot traffic was dense, the path was packed, and it looked like a pedestrian version of a B-road. Parked on the cliff, a Typhoo Tea truck did brisk business. We merged with the flow and headed toward Durdle Door before following the pilgrims down to Lulworth Cove.

§

We stopped at a gas station near Heathrow to fill up the tank. Beverly went into the small market and bought a tube of Superglue. As I topped off the tank, she knelt beside the ravaged tire and glued the flaps of rubber back in place.

"I know it won't last," she said. "But I had to try. It just looked so sad."

At the Avis lot, the inspector came over to evaluate our returned vehicle. First he checked the dashboard and noted that we'd put on 1,512 miles. He asked how we enjoyed our travels and, hearing our American accents, walked directly to the left front corner of the car, bending to study the tire and wheel. He made a few notes.

"Did you hit a pothole?"

The cost wasn't as bad as we'd feared: £130. But we still haven't gotten the final bill for my visit to the doctor, once we got home, for treatment for the rhomboid spasm behind my left shoulder. Apparently, that's not only the muscle used for shifting a British car's standard transmission, it's also—according to my massage therapist and my chiropractor—where I hold my tension.

14

THE FAMOUS RECIPE

Cartwheels on the moon

She might as well have said she had a photograph of my mother turning cartwheels on the moon. Instead, and no less implausibly, Joan said she had a recipe my mother contributed to a cookbook in the late 1950s.

She'd been my brother's fiancée forty-seven years ago, and knew my mother never cooked. She may not have known my mother used the oven as an extra cabinet for stashing pots, pans, platters, and dishes, all wrapped in plastic, but she knew how unlikely it was for her ever to have prepared a dish called *Veal Italienne "Sklootini."*

My mother did, on occasion, make toast. She would open a can of fruit or a container of cottage cheese or jar of jam, cut a chunk of Cracker Barrel cheddar to eat with crackers, pour milk into a bowl of cereal, prepare a cup of instant coffee sprinkled with Sweet'N Low. But the oven and stove as appliances for food production? That was not her world.

She loved to eat, though. She ate slowly, accompanied by dramatic commentary and gesticulations: *Oh! This is divine!* She liked rich, creamy, saucy, elaborate presentations in restaurants, or as a guest at someone else's table, and she wanted everything—from her brandy Alexander through her standing rib roast to her chocolate sundae—amply proportioned. Except on weekends, and provided she didn't have to do the cooking, she didn't seem to mind eating at home, and her preferences remained intact until her death at ninety-five.

One of the last memories I have of my mother comes from a moment a month before she died. Beverly and I were with her as lunch was being served in the solarium of the nursing home's Memory Impairment Unit. Bathed in early spring light, her memory so shattered that she no longer knew who I was or who she herself was, limited to a diet of soft bland food she barely touched, my mother waited for her mushy meal to appear. Though she barely spoke anymore, and never seemed to know where she was, she leaned close to me and said, "The chefs at this restaurant are very, very good."

Lo and behold

Joan also knew, firsthand, about my mother's dedication to disastrous matchmaking, her zeal for bringing ill-suited partners together. This had resulted in my brother's marrying someone else, someone my mother had found for him during his engagement to Joan. Before long, Joan married my basketball coach, without my mother's help, and is still married to him.

We'd lost touch until a few years ago, when we'd begun an e-mail correspondence. Now, she wrote, she'd been "digging deep to find a certain recipe and lo and behold I found a VERY OLD recipe book from The East End Temple Young Married Set and there was a recipe from your mother." I think she understood the startling nature of her discovery, which is why she prefaced it with "lo and behold," as in *You're about to witness the unimaginable!* She concluded by saying the recipe was "very typical of her flamboyant personality," and offered to send me a copy.

The book, mimeographed and plastic comb–bound, was called *130 Famous Long Beach Recipes*. Joan had photocopied the cover and my mother's recipe, which arrived sharing a page with Frieda Schwartz's *Day After Tongue* and Rita Mintz's *Stuffed Cabbage*. I didn't recognize *Veal Italienne "Sklootini"* as something ever served in my home. Or tasted elsewhere. I wondered where she'd found it and why she'd chosen it over such equally fantastical dishes as, say, *Shashlik Sklootovich* or *Chicken Papriskloot*, which we also never encountered.

The recipe itself was like the script for a deadpan Bob Newhart sketch. *You do WHAT to veal scallops? For HOW long? Look, Mrs. Skloot, is this some kind of joke?* It looked and sounded like a recipe, it involved individually credible ingredients, but it read like a spoof.

The very idea of my mother mincing four cloves of garlic, pounding and slicing raw meat, removing the lumps from two cans' worth of Italian tomatoes, or enduring the possibility of tomato stains on the stove struck me as absurd. Then there was the math: two and a half pounds of veal, flattened and cut into two- or three-inch pieces, to be cooked for one hour and fifty minutes. I couldn't imagine what would happen to thin strips of veal cooked that long. And what about the bay leaf listed among the ingredients but never discussed in the cooking directions? Those directions concluded with a serving recommendation: "I suggest that you make spaghetti, to serve an elegant Italian meal, as you will have enough extra sauce."

My mother's recipe had seemed flamboyant to Joan, probably because of its faux French/Italian/Russian name alongside those traditional Jewish recipes for tongue and stuffed cabbage, its assertion of elegance, and the very outlandishness of its existence. But it was my mother's audacity in offering a recipe, when she herself never cooked, that struck me as the wildest, showiest, most characteristic aspect of this magical news.

But I had to wonder if I was remembering right. Did my mother really not cook, as I believed, or was memory deceiving me?

So much as a toothpick

I come from a large family of small families. My father was the third of six siblings who averaged two children each, so we were a dozen cousins, all of us close, visiting on weekends, dining together, celebrating holidays together, going to sleep-away summer camps together.

After learning about Veal Sklootini, I contacted my surviving cousins and asked if they remembered seeing my mother cook. One wrote to say, "We never were at your house for dinner, so that would make me a distant observer on the matter." Another said nearly the same thing: "I don't think I ever ate in your home." What's more, she added, "I truthfully do not remember ever going there." A third wrote that he smiled when he saw the name of the dish, but "I could never imagine her cooking it because I never saw her in the kitchen." He might not be the best person to ask, he said, because—as my other cousins had also said—he didn't "remember spending too much time in your house/home/apartment." A fourth, my oldest cousin, said she didn't even remember our apartment. And a fifth wrote, "I never heard of Lillian lifting so much as a toothpick."

All of us recalled being together and eating together at every other Skloot home. But none recalled eating at ours. Apparently it was accepted that we'd always be dinner guests and never hosts. I don't know how my father and his family reached this level of acceptance or accommodation. Based on what I remember, and what my cousins remember of gatherings at my grandmother's home, or at my aunts' and uncles' homes, for Skloots the kitchen was at the center of life. As I look back across more than half a century, it's difficult to avoid the obvious conclusion: our home had no such center, no place from which the sort of nurturing or comforting or sustaining energy associated with cooking emanated, a locus where everyone gathered and connected and to which everyone was drawn.

To check whether it was just a problem my mother had with my father's family, I contacted other potential witnesses. I called my brother's widow, Elaine, the loving woman he'd found for himself, and lived with through three decades after divorcing the wife my mother had selected for him. Even muffled by the phone, Elaine's laughter when I asked if she'd seen my mother cook startled my cat and made him jump off my lap. "I never saw her do that," she said, eventually. "When we ate with her, which wasn't often, we either went out or she ordered in." Elaine remembers a dinner for six people at my mother's apartment, when all the guests had been told she would be cooking it herself. But my mother had secretly brought the dinner home from a restaurant, a fact revealed when her overcoat, hung hurriedly in the entry closet, was seen to be stained by fresh tomato sauce.

My childhood friend Billy Babiskin remembered the occasional presentation of milk and cookies at my home. "But cooking, NO." He also remembered a parody song his mother and mine created in honor of their culinary preferences. It was sung to the tune of Vincent Youmans's 1929 classic "Without a Song," and their revised lyrics transformed it into a celebration of canned foods: "Without a can, my day would be incomplete / Without a can my family would never eat / Things can't go wrong as long / As you are not without a can." While this may imply they at least heated a can's contents on the stovetop, Billy reiterated that he didn't remember seeing such an act take place in our home. Another childhood friend, Johnny Frank, told me a few years before he died that he never ate in my home. "Eat? I never touched anything in your home." He said he thought of me as "the guy who lived in a museum."

Alice Sachs, wife of the doctor who delivered me in 1947 and who was my godfather, said, "I never saw her cook." Though her husband was among my parents' oldest friends, Alice said, "we were in your apartment maybe twice." Theoretically, she thought, there could have been dinner served, but it wouldn't have been cooked by my mother. "The Princess feeds," Alice said. "Doesn't cook, but feeds."

My stepbrother, Morty, whose father, Julius, had married my mother in 1966, was part of my mother's life for forty years. When I asked if he remembered seeing my mother cook, he said nooooo in a way that combined "of course not" with "is this a trick question?" He also said that "any meals were take-out or eaten in restaurants," and added, "I don't remember her using the oven at all, except for storage." The next day, Morty sent an e-mail elaborating on one particular memory that his wife, Bernice, had mentioned. She remembered eating a chicken that came out of my mother's oven, "but neither of us could remember seeing it go into the oven so it may have been a take-out item. Try as hard as we could, neither of us could remember any other time that we ate anything that had been cooked in that kitchen."

And my daughter, whose memories are freshest, said, "Nope, never saw Grandma cook, not once." She added, "Closest thing I ever saw her do to cooking was once she spread cream cheese on a bagel, which was memorable only because it was the only time I ever saw her do it. That was Julius's job."

The consistency of these responses—even down to the wording— astounded me. I thought I'd find my memory was skewed, or I was exaggerating, and while my mother didn't cook regularly, she'd been seen cooking by *someone*. But no, and it was as though we'd lived in hiding, too.

By the time Beverly and I married in 1993, my twice-widowed mother lived in an apartment in Long Beach and made no pretense of cooking for herself. Dinners were delivered. Food supplies were limited to breakfast and lunch foods whose preparation required nothing more involved than toasting. But when she heard we were coming to Pennsylvania and New York, and bringing Beverly's parents with us, she issued an invitation for Sunday brunch. It would be catered by the Lido Kosher Deli, whose original owners—the Schmaren brothers—had taught me as a teenager to eat hot dogs slathered in slaw instead of sauerkraut. It would also be the first and, it turned out, only meeting between my mother and Beverly's parents. She'd ordered a lavish spread of traditional New York Jewish selections: fresh bagels, cream cheese, two kinds of lox, smoked sable and white fish, herring in sour cream and chopped herring, all surrounded on their platter by an array of lettuce, sliced onion, tomato. My mother was charmed by my tall, handsome father-in-law and he responded to the banquet with delight, saying it was the best he'd ever had. At meal's end, my mother asked if anyone wanted coffee. I knew the correct answer, but unfortunately my in-laws didn't. My mother went into the kitchen and, as the rest of us chatted, I began to worry. After twenty-five minutes had passed, I found her slumped at her small round table in the kitchen, muttering about the *stupid coffee machine*, a thirty-cup percolator for parties, whose operation had been part of Julius's kitchen duties for meetings of the Lions Club. She didn't know how to use the thing, was unwilling to serve my in-laws instant, and, I imagine, was counting on them to forget their desire for coffee. When I asked if she'd like me to make some, she looked away and nodded. There was a can of Maxwell House deep in the cupboard, encased in two large baggies, untouched since Julius's death.

Cook: to prepare food for eating by applying heat

After fourteen hours at his chicken market, my father wanted a home-cooked dinner. And technically, that's what he'd get: His dinner had been cooked at home. It hadn't been prepared by his wife, nor at a time even close to when he ate it, but it had been heated and then reheated in the kitchen in our home.

My father would arrive in the apartment just after seven, put his hat in the hall closet and his cigar in the living room's chrome standing-ashtray, then spend the next five minutes in the bathroom scrubbing his hands. I could hear him blow his nose and hack to clear his throat, getting rid, I believed, of the day's load of feathers and chicken blood. That Nocturne for Faucet and Facial Orifices was the soundtrack to which my mother started and completed her day's food preparation duties: removing whatever was in the oven or on the stovetop and setting it on the table.

Until 1957, when I was ten, we lived in a small, fourth-floor, East Flatbush apartment. Its rent, coupled with the rent on his market, was an ongoing source of worry for my father. *I got the rents, I got the Mafia I'm paying, now I got these supermarkets taking my customers. Where's the money supposed to come from?* We were going broke, he said. But we had a maid. *Just tell me one thing, all right? What is it you do all day that you need a maid?*

I remember our maid vividly. Lassie Lee Price had a warm gap-toothed smile and vast brown eyes, was originally from Alabama, was now living in Brooklyn, and spent seven hours a day in our apartment, arriving at around nine while my mother still slept. Lassie cleaned floors and surfaces that hadn't gotten dirty since she'd cleaned them the day before, changed the bedding, washed and ironed clothes, shopped for groceries, looked after me, and made lunch—which was also my mother's breakfast—and dinner. Since she left our apartment around four, her final act of the day was to prepare a meal that would cook slowly and then sit until the family gathered at seven fifteen to eat it.

My mother had established that certain foods were to be served on certain nights. I know steak was Monday and chicken was Friday, but can't remember the exact schedule for meat loaf or some form of ground meat, for roast beef, for lamb chops. Fish was eaten in restaurants. We seldom had soups and we never had stews or leftovers, which my mother deemed *peasant food*. I remember no cookbooks or discussion of recipes. Preparation was always straightforward: meat was roasted or baked or braised or simmered, any procedure that could take a long time; no sautés or stir-fries, no grilling or broiling, no frills, no fancy brown-then-bake maneuvers, no sauces or gravies. There were canned vegetables, baked potatoes, the occasional slice of bread. It remains inconceivable to me that *Veal Italienne "Sklootini"* could have emerged from our Brooklyn culinary environment. On a Monday, no less.

After my father sold his market, we moved to a rented home in Long Beach and lived on the main floor. The owners occupied a basement apartment during the summer. But little about the way we lived was altered by our move. My father still left home early and returned late, commuting to Manhattan, where he managed the factory floor of my uncle's dress business. And, though Lassie was no longer with us, my mother still had a maid, hiring and losing or firing them until she found Hannah. Slender, brooding, given to vociferous whispers as she zoomed around the house, Hannah was a wizard of efficiency who got along with my mother by saying *yez miz Sloot* and ignoring all but the most basic instructions. There was, apparently, no arguing with Hannah's results, only her process, and my mother kept Hannah with her until my father died, four years later.

Maybe Hannah was responsible for my mother's recipe. I can't be certain, but the cookbook was assembled right around the time she entered our lives. I can imagine my forty-seven-year-old mother coming home from a meeting at the synagogue and sitting in the kitchen to drink a cup of Maxwell House prepared by Hannah, complaining about the ridiculous idea of putting together a cookbook. She wouldn't want to admit she didn't cook, in case that reflected badly on her image as a cultured, refined cosmopolitan woman, the modern woman as an effortlessly gourmet chef. At the same time, she would also not want to admit she did cook, in case that reflected badly on her image as an aristocratic and worldly figure of privilege rather than a kitchen drudge. But if she did contribute a recipe, it would have to be something that stood out from the rest, that showed her to be a culinary sophisticate.

What's the most elegant, epicurean meat? *Veal!* What's the fanciest, priciest cut of veal? *Scallops!* What's the most complex, polished cuisine? *French! Italian!* Ok, then, *Veal Italienne "Sklootini"!* How do you cook that? *Probably just like that brisket you make, Hannah. Yez miz Sloot.*

Rubber sole

From the moment I saw the recipe, I felt I had to cook it. As avid about cooking as my mother was about not cooking, I saw this as a chance to complete something for her. It would be a tribute to her intention, as I understood it, in submitting the recipe, in presenting herself as the kind of person who cooked such a dish. I realized it would also be a gesture symbolic of reclaiming the loving, fortifying, nourishing hearth that had never existed. But I needed some advice first, in case my assumptions about cooking veal scallops were wrong. After all, Beverly and I didn't eat veal, seldom ate red meat of any kind, and had been following a gluten-free diet for the last year and a half.

In *How to Cook Everything*, award-winning food journalist Mark Bittman writes, "Back in the 1950s and 1960s, before we 'discovered' boneless chicken breasts, slices of veal cut from the leg—called *cutlets*, *scallops*, or *scallopine*—were the only thin, tender, boneless meat widely available." Though veal is lean, "properly cooked, it will also be quite tender." Recipes for veal scallopine I found in various cookbooks or online said to cook the flattened meat for one minute per side, then remove it from the pan, pour on the sauce, and serve. I didn't find any recipes that called for browning veal scallops ten minutes per side, then adding ingredients for a sauce and cooking for an additional ninety minutes. It seemed that you might cook certain veal steaks or chops that long, but not flattened, tender scallops. Cut into two- or three-inch pieces.

Beverly checked online and found a recent article from a Washington, D.C.-area magazine, *Flavor*, dedicated to "cultivating the capital foodshed." Focused on the boom in pasture-raised, rose-colored veal, cultivated to replace the inhumanely confined, milk-fed animals whose treatment had driven consumers away, the article mentioned Marcel's Restaurant in Washington's West End, where the chefs were experienced with veal. So I called to speak with Chef Paul about my mother's recipe.

"I would never do that," he said. "If it's good, tender, pounded? No way. No more than four minutes, total."

I asked what he would do with two and a half pounds of veal scallops. He told me to be sure the meat was flattened, and I could hear him begin pounding some hard surface by the phone as he spoke. "Flour it, sear it, maybe with some garlic, and put the meat right on your sauce. Serve it over spinach, that would be nice."

Just before hanging up, I asked Chef Paul what would happen if I followed my mother's recipe. "What will happen? You'll ruin it and you'll waste your money."

I began to wonder if duplicating my mother's recipe was a bad idea. My point wasn't to show that her ideas about cooking were as misguided as her ideas about matchmaking, and I didn't need to cook *Veal Italienne "Sklootini"* to demonstrate that anyway, given how Chef Paul reacted to the recipe.

I called my friend Roger Porter for advice. He teaches English at Reed College here in Portland and was a food critic for the city's daily newspaper, the *Oregonian*. Roger listened to the recipe and assured me the meat would fall apart. He thought for a moment, then said, "But you should cook it, and expense be damned." He offered to split the cost and cook the dish with me. And eat it, if possible. But our schedules didn't match up, and I was still wavering about whether to follow the recipe, so Roger suggested I call Robert Reynolds, founder of the Chef's Studio, a culinary training school in Portland that specializes in French and Italian cooking classes for both professionals and amateurs. "He's the most interesting chef in town." As a final comment, Roger advised me to think of my mother's recipe as "a deathbed command. Her last horrific gift to you." That didn't actually help.

After Robert Reynolds heard my story and my mother's recipe, he said, "You could call it 'Rubber Sole.'" He then told me to throw the results away and take my guests out to dinner. He also thought the recipe wasn't particularly Italian: "It has less to do with Florence than with Prague."

Then Robert made a point that changed everything: it wouldn't be possible for me to duplicate my mother's recipe because I wouldn't be using the same kind of meat. Milk-fed veal, which my mother would have bought in the late 1950s, was white meat. The veal I would buy now, imported from Canada by Whole Foods, is red meat, and completely different in taste, texture, composition, and appearance. "It's young beef, not veal, and they don't compare. You're spared. You can't re-create her dish, so you might as well make something good instead."

He recommended even less cooking than Chef Paul had: thirty seconds on one side, twenty-five on the other. "Then slip it into your sauce to keep warm." If I absolutely had to try my mother's approach, he advised, I should use a cheaper white meat like pork or chicken breast. "But, what would be the point?"

Condensing the universe

Three nights before my mother's one hundredth birthday, I served *Veal Italienne "Sklootini"* to Kerry and Nigel Arkell, friends for more than a quarter century, who have long demonstrated willingness to forgive me for any culinary disaster. Once they'd heard about the recipe's appearance and my discussions with the experts, they volunteered to eat any version I chose to cook.

They arrived with a bottle of claret, a salad, and homemade kale chips, and gathered around the kitchen island. My first thought was that this way of visiting, and this comfort around the cooking zone, was something I treasure, and now I understood more about why that was so. Then I thought it may have been something my mother, in some unexplored recess of her mind, had yearned for but could never pursue because of her class anxieties or aristocratic pretensions or fear of mess. And perhaps that was behind her impulse to submit the recipe for a dish that combined—potentially—basic, homey, one-dish comfort and a certain level of European stylishness: *Veal Italienne "Sklootini."*

I'd made the tomato sauce early in the afternoon and let it simmer for ninety minutes, borrowing the cooking time from my mother's recipe but keeping the veal out of it. The sauce used all my mother's ingredients except the mystery bay leaf, whose use was ignored by the recipe too, but I substituted fresh for canned mushrooms and fresh Italian parsley for dried flakes. It also included a few additions: onions as requested by Beverly, olives as desired by me, basil in honor of Nigel—who is from England and whom I called Basil the first time we met—and red wine because I couldn't imagine tomato sauce without it.

I had water heated for the gluten-free brown rice pasta, a dish with rice flour to coat the veal, and a sauté pan ready on the stove. So there was little left to do except open the wine and drink a toast to my mother.

The final preparations were quick, hectic, and splattery, and I could feel my mother turning away until it would end. When the pasta was finished, I made a mistake, lifting the nestled strainer from the pot while it was still on the stove and sending a cascade of starchy water all over the place. My mother was now officially out of the room, unwilling to be in the presence of such mess. *You see? This is why I didn't cook.* With the drained spaghetti in a serving platter, I poured on the sauce and turned back to the stove. The lightly floured veal got seared for longer than Robert Reynolds's recommended fifty-five seconds but less than Chef Paul's four minutes, and was still pink in the middle when I put it into the sauce and declared the meal ready to eat. My mother came back so we could drink a second toast to her and dig into *Veal Italienne "Sklootini" 2010.*

I wish I'd thought of adding an extra place setting and cup of wine to our table for my mother, as we did during Passover Seders to welcome the prophet Elijah. I could imagine my mother gazing at the heaped platter and nodding, then spreading her arms wide in one of her extravagant dinner-table gestures, declaring the food *divine,* and asking if we expected anything less. What I felt surprised me: a sense of harmony with my mother that would never have been possible in the life I shared with her. It was as though the act of cooking her dish had breached time, had allowed me to reach my mother in ways that had been unimaginable in her life or since her death. I thought of a sentence from one of my favorite cooking-related memoirs, Betty Fussell's *My Kitchen Wars:* "Cooking connects every hearth fire to the sun," she wrote, "and smokes out whatever gods there be—Along with the ghosts of all our kitchens past, and all the people who have fed us with love and hate and fear and comfort, and who we in turn have fed. A kitchen condenses the universe."

Though I'd cut the recipe nearly in half, the four of us couldn't finish all the food. Since Nigel would be on his own for the next few days while Kerry traveled to the Oregon coast, we sent the leftovers home with him. A few days later, I called to ask how *Veal Italienne "Sklootini"* held up over time.

"Very, very well," he said. "I had it two nights in a row, it was good enough for that." This surprised me, since I was sure reheating would toughen the meat. "No, no, I could cut it with a fork." Then, after a pause, he said, "of course, it could just be another Brit happy not bothering to cook, but I liked it even better the next nights."

My mother would have loved Nigel's accent. She would have been pleased to hear that such a sophisticated man appreciated her recipe, exactly the sort of fellow she had in mind to impress. She might even overcome her shock at learning that he would eat leftovers.

🌀

Veal Italienne "Sklootini" 1958

olive oil
1 bay leaf
2½ lbs. veal—flattened & cut into 2- or 3-inch pieces
2 cans Italian plum tomatoes, pressed with fork until almost smooth
salt & pepper
oregano
parsley flakes
1 small can mushrooms (optional)
1 regular or 4 Italian green peppers (remove seeds & cut into slices)

Heat about 5 tbsp. of olive oil & 4 large cloves of garlic (minced) in a large skillet, until garlic is a light golden brown. Add veal & heat on both sides for about 10 minutes. Add 2 large cans of Italian tomatoes (pressed to remove end lumps), salt & pepper, a tsp. of oregano & let simmer for about 90 minutes. Stir several times. 10 minutes before serving, cut in the green pepper & a sprinkling of parsley flakes. You may also add a small can of button mushrooms at the end. I suggest that you make spaghetti, to serve an elegant Italian meal, as you will have enough extra sauce.

Lillian Skloot

Veal Italienne "Sklootini" 2010

(Gluten-Free)
olive oil
1½ lbs. veal scallops
small sweet onion sliced
4 cloves garlic
1 large and 1 small can crushed tomatoes
1 tbsp. tomato paste
1 green pepper, cubed
oregano
basil
fresh Italian parsley, chopped
¼ cup red wine
15–20 pitted Kalamata olives
12–15 fresh mushrooms, sliced
salt & pepper
1 package gluten-free spaghetti (such as brown rice spaghetti)
grated fresh parmesan cheese

Heat olive oil and add onion. As onion softens, add garlic and brown. Add green pepper. Add mushrooms and sauté till mushrooms have given up liquid. Add herbs. Add tomatoes and tomato paste. Then add wine and simmer, covered, for at least 90 minutes. Toss in Kalamata olives.

Prepare spaghetti. Add to platter and top with sauce.

Shortly before serving, heat olive oil in another pan. Coat veal scallops in rice flour. When oil is hot, sear scallops for 30–60 seconds, then turn and sear for another 25–45 seconds. Remove from pan, place in sauce, and serve. Provide grated parmesan cheese on side.

Floyd Skloot